DATE DUE

~~MR 7 '01~~		
~~FE 4 02~~		
~~AP 22 02~~		
~~OC 8 '03~~		
~~FE 1 4 '08~~		

DEMCO 38-296

Dr. Hirsch's Guide to *Scentsational* Weight Loss

Dr. Hirsch's Guide to Scentsational Weight Loss

ALAN R. HIRSCH, M.D.

ELEMENT

Rockport, Massachusetts • Shaftesbury, Dorset
Brisbane, Queensland

ks, Inc. 1997

Text © Alan R. Hirsch, M.D. 1997

First published in the USA in 1997 by
Element Books, Inc.
21 Broadway, Rockport, MA 01966

Published in Great Britain in 1997 by
Element Books Limited
Shaftesbury, Dorset SP7 8BP

Published in Australia in 1997 by
Element Books Limited for
Jacaranda Wiley Limited
33 Park Road, Milton, Brisbane 4064

Library of Congress Cataloging-in-Publication Data

Cover design by Slatter-Anderson
Typeset by Paperwork

Hirsch, Alan R.
  Dr. Hirsch's guide to scentsational weight loss / Alan R. Hirsch
  p. cm.
  Includes appendix.
  1. Weight loss. 2. Aromatherapy. I. Title
RM222.2 H56 1997
613.2'5—dc20   96-41203
                                                     CIP

British Library Cataloguing in Publication data available
Abstract is reprinted by permission of *The Journal of Neurological and
Orthopedic Medicine and Surgery* (1995) 16:26-31
First Edition

10 9 8 7 6 5 4 3 2 1

Printed and bound by Edwards Brothers, Inc., Michigan, USA
ISBN 1–85230–950–4

Contents

*To my wife, Debra,
and our two children,
Marissa and Jack, and to
the thousands of people
who helped us demonstrate
that this new idea for
weight control does work*

Foreword

I have had the pleasure of knowing Dr. Alan Hirsch for more than twenty years. We both entered medicine while teenagers as part of the Inteflex Program, a six-year combined undergraduate and medical school program at the University of Michigan, and that time together has produced a friendship that has lasted more than half of my life

Alan was a year behind me. I soon found he was indeed unique. He was intelligent, creative, funny, and always interesting. In the entire time that I have known him, I've never spent a boring moment when he was around.

School was hard work, but Alan and I had a good time. We crashed down a hill on a tandem bicycle (end over end) without getting hurt. We used a real screw to uncork a bottle of wine (semi-successfully). We went swimming in a beautiful hotel pool without being registered guests. Alan, Steven (his brother), and I spent ten hours (for a four-hour trip) on an Amtrak train traveling from Ann Arbor to Chicago during a giant snowstorm and didn't suffer a bit. I also remember enjoying lavish dinners we really couldn't afford during birthday celebrations (our birthdays are a day apart). To work those dinners off, we ran on a track (he ran; I jogged). We studied in the library and hoped that the good-looking girls would notice us (once in a while they even did).

Several years later my wife, Cathie, met Alan and his wife, Debra, for the first time. I was afraid that if she didn't like them, my longtime friendship would be jeopardized. Fortunately, Cathie immediately appreciated the vitality this amazing duo has, helping strengthen the bonds of our important friendship.

Alan was a fine student. He has been interested in neurology and psychiatry for as long as I can remember. Typical of his dedication to patient care, he spent a summer (as a student) caring for the needs of aphasic patients (those with speech disorders after stroke or brain injuries) while they underwent intensive speech therapy. As befits his remarkable creativity, he has now found a unique niche working with and studying the sense of smell. I was aware of his busy practice and scholarly publications for a long time. I was not aware that news of his interesting work had reached the general public until recently. While at home on vacation, my wife yelled to me. "Guess who is on 'Oprah'!" When I was told it was Alan, I ran quickly to the set. He was, as usual, interesting and funny. However, I was also struck by how informative he was and by how many people could benefit from knowledge of his work. I have since learned that he has appeared on numerous TV and radio shows including "20/20," "48 Hours," "The Today Show," "Jerry Springer," "Dateline," "Beyond 2000," and "Good Morning America." He has also done research for major industrial powers.

In August of 1996, Alan and I were talking on the phone. He mentioned that he was preparing a new book about using the sense of smell to help control weight. I was interested in the subject, and we talked about it for a while. He then asked me if I would be interested in writing the foreword to the book. I am normally skeptical of "self-help" publications, but I agreed to have a look at his manuscript. I started reading and was immediately captivated. The book style is so comfortable. You feel as if you are in Dr. Hirsch's office and he is sitting with you and quietly discussing the rationale for his technique. Patient-oriented examples throughout the book also enhance its genuine quality. To be sure, the science of the brain is complicated, but it is explained so simply and clearly that it is easy for someone without any background to understand. The topics chosen such as "Diets Don't Work," "Rebounding," and "Our Emotions Can't Be Ignored," are perfectly suited to people struggling with their weight. Unlike many books where the concept sort of fades into oblivion, this book ends in a bang with "Ask Away!" This final chapter packs a wallop and keeps you interested until the very last word.

I am honored that I was asked to write the foreword to *Dr. Hirsch's Guide to Scentsational Weight Loss*. Readers everywhere will be delighted to read this *sensational* book. It is certainly a practical, biological approach to an important health problem.

Like any close friends, Alan and I share some thoughts that are unique to our relationship. Therefore, in closing, I must say "bionicism forever"—my friend, you have written a terrific book.

RICHARD TROHMAN, M.D.
DEPARTMENT OF CARDIOLOGY
CLEVELAND CLINIC
OCTOBER 1996

Preface

You are about to read a book that in my wildest dreams I couldn't have imagined writing. Only a few years ago, I knew almost nothing about dieting and the lifelong struggles to lose weight experienced by so many people. One could say that my interest in the role of odors in promoting weight loss happened by accident.

As a neurologist and psychiatrist, I developed an interest in olfaction (the sense of smell) from treating patients who had lost their sense of smell because of illness, side effects of medications, head trauma, and so forth. I noted that many of my patients had actually gained weight once their sense of smell was impaired. It's as if they overate in an attempt to regain some of the pleasure from eating that had been lost along with the sense of smell. Since 90 percent of taste is really smell, if we can't smell food, we don't taste it. So these people were consuming more food but most certainly enjoying it less—it's difficult, if not impossible, to enjoy food that has no taste.

It's true that some people actually lose weight when their sense of smell is impaired because they lose interest in food—they may even forget to eat. But so many other people keep on eating and don't understand why they actually consume more food when they can't smell or taste it.

As you will learn as you read this book, a physiological connection exists between the odor of food and the center in the brain, the satiety center, that tells us that we've eaten enough. This led me to believe that it was possible that the sense of smell could be called on to actually help people lose weight. Perhaps, I thought, our new knowledge about the sense of smell would help us design a weight loss program that marshaled the power of smell. We could work with the body, not against it, to help people consume less food, but without a formal "diet."

When we started this research, I knew almost nothing about diets. But they all seemed based on specific food plans and every one involved restriction and led to feelings of deprivation. The research I did told me that diets don't work—at least not in a lasting way. This is a tragic situation because obesity is one of the primary health problems affecting adults—and children—in our society. As if that weren't bad enough, overweight people are fighting against evolution and against genetics. They are scorned in our society, and they are among the most courageous people I've ever met—our research with more than three thousand people taught me about the ugly prejudice they are subjected to. If we can use the sense of smell to improve people's lives, then it is important research indeed.

The best thing about losing weight by using odors is that it is safe as well as effective. There are no drugs to take and no surgeries to undergo. Even if our study had not produced positive results, I knew that the odors would not cause harm to our participants.

This book results from the weight loss and odor study conducted by The Smell and Taste Treatment and Research Foundation, located in Chicago, Illinois. Our foundation has been in existence for more than a decade, and we have three primary missions. The first is to treat patients with smell and taste disorders, and the second is to investigate the effects of odors on mood states and behavior. We have published more than one hundred medical and scientific articles and have presented our findings at more than two hundred national and international meetings. Currently, we have more than eighty-five active studies, which are investigating the effects of odors on exercise, sexual arousal, insomnia, learning, headaches, claustrophobia, agoraphobia, consumer behavior, and productivity.

In this book, you'll read about the many people who lost weight and have kept it off; some participants lost well over 100 pounds. Some people had much less weight to lose, and they too succeeded. Throughout this book I've shared (anonymously) their experiences and comments because I'm certain that if you have battled a weight problem throughout your life, you will identify with our participants' words. I will always be grateful to the men and women who were willing to, once again, embark on a weight loss plan. After all the negative experiences many had been through, they had every reason to be skeptical, but they agreed to work with us, skepticism and all. As the results came in, we at the foundation were extremely pleased, but no one could have been more pleased than the participants.

You are embarking on an exciting adventure—one that most people have never heard of, let alone tried. I urge you to keep an open mind and put the information into action immediately. Like our patients, you too can lose unwanted pounds and keep them off by using your sense of smell as your partner in weight control. Nothing could be more natural than that.

ALAN R. HIRSCH, M.D.
CHICAGO, ILLINOIS

THE ODOR DEVICES: Availability and Warning Statement

Odor devices are widely available nowadays, but our foundation does not endorse specific products. However, at the time of this writing, we are still in the process of evaluating the efficacy of various types on the market. It is our hope that by the time you receive this book, more current data will be available. If you would like information, please write or call:

> The Smell and Taste Treatment
>   and Research Foundation
> Water Tower Place, #990 West
> 845 N. Michigan Avenue
> Chicago, Illinois 60611
> (312) 938-1047

Callers in the UK please dial 0345 023905

Warning: Those who suffer from asthma should *not* use the odor devices. Individuals who get migraine headaches that are triggered by odors also should refrain from using the odor devices, unless they know which specific odors to avoid and which are safe. Anyone attempting to lose weight should be under the care of a physician, who may offer additional advice.

Acknowledgements

A special thanks to the always-hard-working staff at the Smell and Taste Treatment and Research Foundation in Chicago, Illinois, for their daily efforts to advance research on olfaction. And thanks, too, to the administrative and research staff of Mercy Hospital and Medical Center in Chicago. Their support allowed this project to come to fruition. I'd also like to thank Virginia McCullough for her help in seeing this project through to completion and Roberta Scimone of Element Books for recognizing the value of this book.

Many of my colleagues and friends have supported my research endeavors. To name a few would mean leaving out too many, so I offer my appreciation to them as a group, with special mention of Dr. Ervin Hawrylewicz and Dr. Sally Freels of the University of Illinois School of Public Health, and to Stan Block, a true friend.

Family members have been patient and indulgent as I pursued this and other work. A special thanks to Debra for her tolerance and understanding.

Dr. Hirsch's
Guide to
Scentsational
Weight Loss

1 The Dismal Truth: Diets Don't Work

Betts* was only thirty-two, but she'd already lost and gained about 600 pounds over a dozen years in diet programs—wasted years, as far as she and I are concerned. Now, feeling like a complete failure as a person, she was again almost 100 pounds overweight and was preparing to make one more attempt to lose these excess pounds. But rather than feeling excited by the prospect of entering a study that offered a possible new solution to her problem, she was angry and hostile. "So, tell me," she said sarcastically, "about all the foods I *can't* have."

"This isn't a diet," I said. "We all know that diets don't work. Our program is different—very different. But trust me, you won't completely understand how it works until you try it." I went on to explain to Betts that our approach to weight loss was neither based on a special diet nor did it include a list of "forbidden" foods. These guidelines surprised everyone who entered our weight loss/olfaction (smell) study or who have now chosen to use their noses to fight obesity. Given the high failure rate of diets, it's no wonder that Betts, and untold numbers of people like her, view any discussion of a new approach to weight reduction with suspicion.

However, several thousand people have now overcome their skeptical attitude and have accepted that no, diets

Names of all study participants and patients have been changed to protect their privacy.

don't work, but sniffing pounds away does. Before these people could accept that this new system can work, they needed to have some understanding about why their previous attempts to lose weight had failed.

Without question, we can say that over the long term, diets almost never work, but the fault may not lie with the dieter—and that, it appears, is something that most overweight people don't know. For at least part of the reason why, we can look to our evolution.

Millions of Years of Evolution

At any point in time, one third of adult women and one quarter of adult men in the United States meet the medical criteria for a diagnosis of obesity. This makes obesity one of the most pervasive health problems in our society. It has physical and psychological consequences that have an impact on the afflicted in countless ways. If you are reading this book, you may be all too familiar with the suffering I'm talking about.

When I use the word "afflicted," I intend to imply that an obese person is a "victim." While I don't expect an overweight person to be happy about being a victim of *evolution*, I hope this information will help put the rampant problems of obesity in perspective. And, in this case, being afflicted with a problem also means being a *survivor* in a long evolutionary struggle. When I say long, I'm talking about millions of years of the human struggle to survive; and, for much of our history, the quest for survival was a daily concern.

Think about this concept for a minute. When you studied history, did you ever read about a society with not only an abundance of food, but vast stores of *excess* food? You didn't read about such a society because it has never existed before. We are at a unique point in history, and from what we know about human development, this excess of food is actually an unnatural condition.

Most of our ancestors had to accumulate fat in the food-growing season in order to survive cold winters, during which they consumed whatever stored food was available, and when that ran out, they foraged for more. These were the only available options. Until very recently, it was common for food supplies to dwindle during the cold, winter months, particularly in the Northern Hemisphere. Many people became hungry before winter's end, and spring was greeted with great rejoicing, not just because it was warm and pleasant, but because food supplies could be renewed. It's likely that the spring rituals and festivals originated precisely because new plant and animal life appeared just in time to ensure survival for one more year.

We know that it's easier to lose weight in the summer when fat is, in a biological sense, not so necessary because food is available. In the Northern Hemisphere, we developed in a way similar to the black bear; we accumulate fat in the winter as a supplementary source of calories for use when food is scarce.

In the past, periodic famine was not just an occasional threat, it was a regular reality throughout the world. And, during those miserable periods, only those who had stored body fat survived. In fact, those whose bodies could efficiently accumulate fat were strong enough to flourish and reproduce. This is one of the best examples we can look to that demonstrate the principle of "the survival of the fittest." Perhaps when we hear people admire a plump baby, we are also hearing an attitude that has carried over from our evolutionary past. Imagine how relieved new parents were when a baby was born with what at one time was viewed as a positive feature—fat, plenty of fat. Throughout Western literature we can read the descriptions of fat babies and the way in which this was viewed as a sign of good health and a strong constitution.

To be sure, in many places in the world famine is still a reality and threatens to become even more severe.

(Unfortunately, hunger and lack of adequate nutrition is not completely unknown in our own wealthy country either.) One need only look at the nightly news to grasp the fact that only the very strong and constitutionally hardy make it through the periods when getting enough food is the biggest challenge individuals face.

In other countries food scarcity is more than the distant memory it is to most of us born and raised in this country. Indeed, food still is so scarce some places that the main occupation of men and women is securing enough of it to stay alive. Edward, one of our study participants, who has struggled with his weight problem for fifty years, described this paradoxical situation well. "When I lived and worked in a number of Asian countries," he said, "older women in the villages admired my big waistline. They thought I must be prosperous to be so fat. They found Americans fascinating in part because we have these excess pounds. To these women who had been poor most of their lives, my fat was a sign of good fortune—I was blessed with more than enough food."

While a scanty food supply is no longer as pressing an issue in most of the countries Edward worked in, the older people remember the days when famine constantly threatened. And, as we've seen recently in China, food shortages always threaten. It goes without saying that people in many other cultures consider our society's obsession with weight as rather odd and even self-indulgent. While it may be small com-fort if you live in the image-conscious United States, being very thin is not admired in much of the rest of the world.

Ironically, as soon as Edward moved back to the United States, he embarked on numerous diets and even fasting programs in order to lose his excess pounds. Much of the time, he did lose weight, but within a few months he gained the unwanted pounds back—and more. When he first began his quest to lose weight and tried many diets, he had 45 pounds to lose; when I saw him that number had grown to

THE DISMAL TRUTH: DIETS DON'T WORK

more than 100. Predictably, he was unhappy and frustrated.

One African-American woman questioned the premise about fat accumulation in the Northern Hemisphere. After all, she said, her ancestors were not from Europe. Why was she fat? I could tell her only that the distribution of obesity throughout our population suggests that when food becomes plentiful, the evolutionary mandates for survival can lead to excess fat accumulation in all racial groups. This, com-bined with our society's emphasis on food, sets up a situation in which large numbers of people from all racial and ethnic backgrounds become vulnerable to weight gain. We have seen that it takes only a generation or two for weight to become a problem among our immigrant populations.

Fighting Evolution

It's a paradox, but now that the strongest have survived because their ancestors stored fat so efficiently, the problems new generations face have changed. Many people have bodies that are too efficient, and they have a difficult time adapting to our unique conditions, specifically, abundant food all year round. In other words, for many people, the struggle to survive has been won, and now the struggle to maintain health is in conflict with innate biological program-ming and instincts. The body simply doesn't know what is going on here. It's as if it's saying, "Wait a minute here. I'm supposed to be storing fat so that you can get through lean periods. But you're eating so much all year round, and I don't know how to turn this storage system off. What do you want from me? My main job is to make sure you survive, but you're confusing me."

Our bodies are beautifully programmed to maintain homeostasis, that is, to stay the same. Again, this is an im-portant evolutionary strength. When food is scarce, the body will slow the metabolic rate in order to "hoard" its available fuel. The brain gets used to, or set at, a certain weight; it struggles to keep the body stabilized at that weight, usually referred to as the "set point." Fortunately, the set point can be changed, a topic I'll discuss in chapter 8.

The yo-yo syndrome is the result of the body's fight to maintain homeostasis. If diets worked, then each overweight person would go on one diet in a lifetime and never need to worry about the scale traveling up and down—again and again. But, we're in a situation in which it appears that homeostasis, the evolutionary friend, has now become the dieter's enemy.

It's no wonder that the majority of people in our studies had not only been on numerous self-directed diets, they had also participated in many commercial or employer-sponsored weight loss programs. Astounding as it seems, our participants listed close to one hundred different pro-grams. Every person had been on at least six or seven diets before entering our weight loss program. In almost every case, the weight returned in a relatively short period of time—sometimes within a few months.

Many overweight people complain about the frustrating plateaus of weight loss they experience while dieting. We can explain these as simply part of the process of homeostasis, but that seldom relieves the stress that dieters feel when their best efforts are not rewarded. Yet, for its own very good reasons, having to do with its instinct to survive, the body will respond to reduced calories by attempting with even more vigor to maintain its energy stores.

The yo-yo syndrome is most dramatic among people who fast or who are on the very-low-calorie diets. Some people cut their calorie intake even more during a plateau, which leads to lack of energy and increased hunger. Even-tually, most people stop the diet, usually believing that they have failed again. It's difficult enough to lose weight when you feel good, but when you feel physically and emotionally defeated, it is almost impossible. As you will see in chapter 7, using odors to improve your mood and enhance well-being is part of this weight loss system if you choose to use it.

Women Are Most Affected on the Evolutionary Trail

You've no doubt heard women say, "It's so infuriating. He eats one piece of toast instead of two, switches to light beer, cuts his snacks in half, and he loses weight. I practically starve myself to get rid of one lousy pound, and he's boasting about the five pounds he's dropped this week. I can't stand it."

Back to evolution. In the interest of survival of our species, women are extremely important. Much as we men may dislike this, it's a fact that in the natural scheme of things, nature can afford to lose more men than women. So, women who can store enough fat to not only survive, but to reproduce too, are the hardiest among us.

Unfortunately, this biological imperative also makes it difficult for women to lose weight, particularly premenopausal women whose fertility must, in the evolutionary sense, be protected. A husband can brag about his weight loss, but in our abundant society, he now has a distinct advantage. The fact that he's more biologically dispensable makes it easier for him to fight evolution. This is one reason more women are overweight than men.

Estrogen, one of the female hormones responsible for ovulation, also appears to play a part in maintaining weight. Where once this was a blessing, it is now a curse of sorts. Back when food supplies were seasonal and generally scarce, a woman who efficiently maintained body fat could ovulate and carry a fetus to term. Hence, regeneration could continue because of women's ability to store fat and because of the body's struggle to maintain homeostasis.

Frankly, our bodies haven't changed much in response to excess food supplies. In our weight loss study, we noted that premenopausal women, and those on estrogen replacement therapy (ERT), lost weight at a slower rate than men of all ages and postmenopausal women who were not taking estrogen. (This difference should not discourage women from attempting to lose weight with this smell-device program, nor should it prompt them to stop taking estrogen. Many women benefit from ERT in that it may help prevent osteoporosis and symptoms associated with menopause. The relative benefits and risks of ERT should be discussed with your gynecologist.)

The biological situation, which works against women, combined with our society's emphasis on being thin, contribute to the continuation of the yo-yo syndrome. More diets, more self-help programs, more weight loss centers. And for many people, especially women, this atmosphere finally results in the depressing conclusion that one more diet isn't the answer. But the answer is the same for men, too. Diets simply don't work.

It's Just Not Fair

If you get the feeling that you've been set up to struggle with weight, and that it just doesn't seem fair, you're entirely correct. You may be like many of the more than three thousand people in our major weight loss study; you've gained and lost hundreds of pounds in your lifetime; you've suffered from the emotional roller coaster that goes along with yo-yo dieting; perhaps you've suffered serious consequences, both physical and emotional, from being overweight.

In addition to fighting evolution, you are also up against society's emphasis on food—coexisting with worshiping thinness, a trend that is especially popular right now. Just think about the food messages that daily bombard you and urge you to eat. Both the sight and smell of food are before us constantly, ever enticing us to eat more and more; "all you can eat" is a watchword of some restaurants and even in some of our homes. We are programmed to think that there is never enough, and more is better. (Of course, this "more is better" mentality affects practically everything from food to the amount of money we make to the size of our homes. It can be a discouraging mind-set; it may feed our competitive drive, but is ultimately demoralizing for so many people.)

In addition to the temptations that surround us, most overweight people acknowledge that they also use food for comfort. The mere act of eating can relieve stress and inner turmoil. Yet, many of those who are not overweight eat for the same reasons. People in our society joke about eating ice cream when they don't have a date on Saturday night. Or, people freely talk about overeating at dinner on the day the big business deal fell through. However, it's usually the thin people who banter about this openly; the overweight person often keeps silent or will attempt to deny that he or she uses food to combat emotional difficulty. They some-times think of this as a secret shame, and only in support groups will they "confess" to overeating—even binging—when they feel sad or hopeless.

Later in this book (chapter 7), you'll learn more about the link between food and emotional well-being. While eating for emotional reasons has often been viewed as a problem or, in some cases, a serious emotional disorder, the fact is it is a nearly universal phenomenon. Overweight people aren't really very different from their slimmer sisters and brothers.

The vast majority of people have used food for purposes other than to meet nutritional needs. When we were babies, we cried and were offered food as comfort—maybe we were hungry and maybe we weren't. In either case, we associated this offer of food with love and being taken care of. As children, we may have been rewarded with food when we got good grades or when our family was celebrating some event. Sybil, a participant in our study, told us that her family had an elaborate dinner in an expensive restaurant every time her mother sold one of her paintings. Clearly, food was associated with success, and is it any wonder that now, when Sybil makes an important sale for her company, her first impulse is to eat? (When she loses a sale, her urge to eat is just as strong.) Her emotional response is learned behavior.

Martin found that when he was following one of his strict diets, it was difficult to have a social life. Women he dated didn't understand that he wanted to skip dinner and head straight to the movie theater. His dates didn't particularly like it when he didn't want to share a bucket of buttered popcorn and he preferred not to be tempted at a café where good-smelling pastries called out to him from display cases. So ingrained is our association of food with sociability that Martin ended up isolated when he found it too difficult to handle constant temptation. Because diets don't work anyway, Martin went through periods of having a social life, with all the associated meals and treats, alternating with periods of being alone, combined with attempts to lose weight. Believe me, his yo-yo story is not unique.

I've heard people say that they were urged not to start a diet until after the holidays—after all, how could they enjoy the season between late November and January unless they could eat, eat, eat? Others have said that they are afraid of hurting a relative's feelings by not taking second helpings of some holiday delicacy. Literally hundreds of reasons are used to justify eating more than we should, and the overweight aren't the only people pulling them out of the hat when needed.

So, if you are overweight and sense that the cards have been stacked against you, you are right. And it isn't fair. In addition to having biological factors working against you, you also have against you the very society that urges you to eat.

The Last Great Prejudice

I want to make it clear that I am not a "diet doctor." I am a neurologist who is also a psychiatrist. I became interested in olfaction while I was still in medical school, after I temporarily lost my sense of smell following a head injury resulting from an accident on my bicycle. These many years later, my research on our sense of smell has taken me in many directions, from odors and consumer buying habits to odors and sexuality, and much more. Using smell as an aid to weight loss is just one of the many projects our foundation has undertaken. Some of the information has crossover application. For example, you'll learn more about scents that reduce anxiety and how they might be useful to you as you sniff pounds away.

My professional practice has primarily been focused on treating people who have lost their sense of smell. For this reason, I was not completely aware of the deep-seated and ugly prejudice in our society against overweight people. In fact, I came to realize that it is probably the last "allowable" bias. While stereotyping of African-Americans, Hispanics, Jews, women, or homosexuals is considered ignorant, stereotyping the overweight is still acceptable. Jokes can be made about obese people that would not be tolerated about any other group; *judgments* can be made about the very character of overweight people that would sound completely ridiculous if made about persons in other groups. While we would never call any other group of people lazy, this is the most common judgment made against the obese in our society.

Almost all overweight people suffer derision and ridicule, but the worst prejudice is reserved for and directed toward obese women. We need only look at television commentators, politicians, and others in public life to realize that overweight men do not experience the same degree of discrimination that obese women suffer. (It's no exaggeration to say that obese women are, as one of my patients put it, "society's pariahs.") I've even heard overweight husbands belittle their wives for gaining weight. When challenged, one such husband declared, "Extra pounds don't matter so much for a man. A woman has to be thin to be attractive." It took several decades and even some lawsuits to modify the ridiculous weight requirements instituted by many airlines for their flight attendants.

Some women in our study expressed the belief that others wished they didn't exist. "It's as if I don't have the same right to live," one woman said, after describing one especially insulting incident in which an airline passenger complained of having to sit next to her for a ninety-minute flight. Another patient added, "You can't imagine what it's like to have people take away your food in a restaurant, as if they are doing you a favor by punishing you like a child. Don't they know we need food to live, too?" This false belief that the overweight person doesn't need food can lead the obese to try destructive fasts, which almost always lead to still more weight gain.

Those who would continue their prejudice should think about the endless struggle against evolution that overweight people face—and very few haven't tried to fight this battle many times. Basic biology works against the notion that we must all be thin. Oddly, the ideal person is thought to be one who is tall and thin. But when we look at the world's population, we can see that most of us are simply not programmed to fit this image.

Perhaps most important of all, the prejudice against the overweight has serious psychological consequences. Eight percent of our study participants expressed a desire to kill themselves—at that time, not just at some point in the past. Over three quarters of the people believed themselves to be ugly or unattractive; about a third of the group had lost interest in other people; over a third said they were sad most or all of the time. In large numbers, this group of people expressed extreme dislike for themselves, hopelessness for the future, and guilty feelings about their bodies and their past failures to lose weight. They spoke about being tired all the time, missing at least one day of work a month because of weight-related problems, lack of interest in sex, and ongoing depression. (The majority tested positive for clinical depression.)

I realize, of course, that the group I'm talking about is composed of people who were seriously concerned about their weight and had social, medical, and emotional consequences from their obesity. They sought help—again—because they wanted to change their lives. Some overweight people have made a good adjustment to their situation and are not held back in life by their weight. People in this group would, by necessity, have had to successfully ignore the discrimination that is directed against them. But this doesn't make the discrimination fair or right. Prejudice against the overweight is both mean-spirited and ignorant, just as it is when it's directed to any other group. As I worked with our study participants, I came to realize this more and more. I also understand what great courage it takes to tackle the problem of being overweight, which is now a pervasive health problem.

Motivation and Action

The difficulties of losing weight and the prejudice against the obese notwithstanding, most people with weight problems will continue to become motivated to try to reach a normal weight. Because you are reading this book, you are probably one of those people. And so, as you begin to learn how your sense of smell can be used to affect your appetite and weight in a positive way, bear in mind that the information you encounter is not the makings of a new diet. You will not even use the word diet when you think or talk about this program. I have no list of forbidden foods, although I do offer some suggestions about healthful eating in chapter 9. You won't be given a list of foods you must eat at breakfast or at lunch; you will not be weighing your foods or counting calories. You don't have to shop at special stores and you can eat in restaurants without asking that the food be prepared in a special way just for you.

As you will see in this book, which discusses the role of your sense of smell in weight loss, you have many tools to use as you struggle to lose weight in this program—the most important one being odor devices. We'll discuss ways you can use these odor devices when you wake up in the morning or when you go to bed at night; you'll learn to use them at work, in restaurants, at a friend's home, in movie theaters, or even on the train as you go to work. We'll also talk about the role odors can play to balance your moods and improve your concentration; you'll also learn how the timing and frequency of meals can enhance this program. In addition, I'll offer some information about food cravings and addictions and some tips to overcoming these problems.

Before you can effectively use odors as a weight loss aid, you need to understand why this system works so well. Both physiology (the way the body works) and psychology are involved in making this program a success, but for now, we'll start at the beginning, with that marvelous feature, your nose.

2 Sniff to Lose Weight— But Why?

"If food wasn't so appealing," Barry said, "I wouldn't want to keep eating. Is there any way that food can be made so unpleasant that I'd just stop eating when I feel full—or better yet, eat only enough to get the calories I need but not be tempted to eat more?" Barry's question is quite common. When people ask it, they do so with a sincere desire to stop eating so much food in order to lose weight. Like many people, Barry believed that the pleasure inherent in eating was the primary cause of his overeating and his excess pounds. He was like so many overweight people, in that he associated taking pleasure in eating with being "bad." Therefore, if food was made to taste awful, he wouldn't eat so much and he might feel better about himself. That would probably be true, for a day or two, but the primary consequence of such a "diet" is generally to drop it quickly and write it off as another failure.

Eating is a pleasurable act and is an integral part of nature's survival plan. If we had no sensation of thirst, we wouldn't survive; if sex weren't inherently pleasurable, we wouldn't engage in it and procreate. If we didn't feel hungry and drawn to eat, our species would rapidly become extinct. We must eat to live, and it's only in this abundant society that our biological mechanisms are disturbed and that now many of us reverse the order, and live to eat.

Keep in mind that all our senses are designed to help us survive. We hear sounds that alert us to danger or that inform us about situations we must cope with in the world around us. We see things that can threaten us, and the same sense allows us to assess the danger and move quickly to a safer place. Our sense of touch alerts us to bodily injury through the mechanism of pain. If we didn't have it, we'd probably die in infancy from self-inflicted injury. Of course, these same senses allow us to hear beautiful music, see a spectacular sunset, and enjoy a soothing massage. Yes, we can adapt to loss or impairment of any of these three senses, but as we all know, it's not easy.

Our two other senses, the ability to smell and taste, are also part of our human survival mechanism, and both senses also bring us great pleasure. The ability to smell and taste spoiled, rotten food also keeps us from poisoning ourselves. Barry may wish to have the mechanism altered, but nature is smarter than our momentary desires.

When we treat patients who experience loss of smell, and consequently have diminished ability to taste, we notice that they often tend to gain weight, not lose it. When they begin to regain their sense of smell (usually through the use of special medications), they start losing their extra pounds. This observation led us to explore the role of smell in appetite and weight control, and the questions we posed resulted in our first study. But before we can under stand how using smells can help with appetite and weight reduction, we must understand how smell is connected to our sense of hunger and to the amount of food we consume.

It Starts in Your Brain

It's a common lament: "If I even see a plate of food, I gain weight," says the overweight person. And it may be that the joke is so common, it seems to be true. But, perhaps it isn't the sight of the food that causes the overindulgence, it's the aroma that causes the conditioned response. Sometimes we smell food, we salivate, and then we believe we're hungry. (Sounds like the proverbial Pavlov's dogs' conditioned response, and it is—more on that in chapter 10.) On the other hand, people who work around food all day often report losing interest in it. The job at the chocolate factory may not be the exciting experience it's reputed to be. It appears that an odor that makes us want to eat when we first detect it eventually loses its appeal.

The mechanism of hunger and feeling full or satisfied is not as simple as it seems. Most of us believe that feeling satisfied is a mechanism that's centered in the stomach, because that's the way we experience it. If you ask people, overweight or not, why they stop eating, they usually respond by saying they get up from the dinner table because they feel full. But this is rarely true. With the exception of big holiday dinners—Thanksgiving, for example, when we do eat until we feel stuffed—we rarely stop eating because we actually have a full stomach.

Some people believe they eat to raise their blood sugar levels. They think their blood sugar is low when they are hungry and that it returns to normal when they've eaten enough. They associate an increase in blood sugar level with their sense of feeling full and satisfied. But this isn't true either. Unless you have reactive hypoglycemia or diabetes, your blood sugar level is the same when you stop eating as it was when you first sat down to enjoy a meal.

In reality, we feel full or satisfied because of a special mechanism in our brain. Specifically, the satiety response is regulated in what is technically known as the ventromedial nucleus of the hypothalamus, a portion of the brain that regulates many basic drives. We call this portion of the hypothalamus the satiety center.

One reason we stop eating is that this center signals a fullness or a sense of being satisfied. It says, "I'm full, I should stop eating now" or "I've had enough of this food," and the fork is put down and the plate taken away. We know that this center works because when it is damaged the mechanism no longer sends its protective signal that tells us to put the fork down. If we damage the satiety center in a hamster, for example, the hamster will eat—and eat and eat—until it dies. It doesn't know when to stop because it has no sensation of fullness.

But what does this have to do with smell? When odor molecules are in the air, they are directed to the olfactory bulb. This bulb is connected to the satiety center in the hypothalamus—an obvious example of nature's careful design. Assuming that the mechanism is working well, the brain can correlate the amount of food that you have taken into your mouth with the amount of odor that has reached the nose. In other words, the satiety center uses the odor molecules to operate its signals of, "You've eaten enough, you are satisfied now." The message might actually be, "I've smelled it, therefore I've eaten it."

Some of our study participants wanted to understand in greater detail how the odors affect the satiety center and the way odors in the air reach the brain. In the following sections of this chapter, I will provide information about the physiology of smell to help answer questions you might have. You could live your whole life without knowing how the mechanism of olfaction works and still enjoy the scents around you. Many of our study participants lost a significant amount of weight without understanding exactly how it works. But, by having this foundation, I hope that you'll gain an understanding of the reasons why I'm asking you to think of your sense of smell as your partner and ally in weight loss.

Feeling Full Starts with Breathing

We seldom notice our breathing, but we inhale and exhale thousands of times each day. We take each breath automatically and rarely think about it, except perhaps when our breathing is labored because we are ill or when we become aware of a strong odor. We might hold our breath and try not to inhale too deeply if we detect an unpleasant odor, such as exhaust fumes from a passing car. This is one way we attempt to protect ourselves from toxic fumes. On the other hand, when we detect an especially appealing scent, such as the smell of lilacs in the spring, we may purposely breathe more deeply to enrich the experience. It's one of life's pleasures.

When we inhale, odor molecules enter a nostril, and normally, the air descends to the lungs. When air currents develop in the nose, the molecules are able to reach the epithelia in the olfactory—or smell—center in the top of the nose, just behind the bone we call the bridge of the nose. The epithelia are protective, mucous-coated membranes about the size of a shirt button or a dime.

I like to think of these air currents as small gales or tornadoes that develop because we inhale deeply. Odd as it might seem, these strong air currents develop when the nose is partially stuffed up. (When the nose is totally stuffed up, then the ability to smell is reduced. We've all had this experience when we've had a cold.) Furthermore, our olfactory ability depends on which nostril is open and which is closed. Although you seldom notice it, both nostrils are not equally open or closed at any given time. In fact, one is usually open while the other is closed, and in the normal course of things, this changes every eight hours or so. We call this the olfactory cycle.

You can test the olfactory cycle for yourself. Put your index finger over one side of the nose to close the nostril and then inhale. Close the other side of the nose and inhale again. One nostril will be more open than the other—or more stuffed up than the other. You'll actually have better olfactory ability in the nostril that's more stuffed up.

An odor molecule in the air makes its way to the top of the nose to a pin-sized area of the olfactory membrane where millions of olfactory receptors are found. The odor molecule moves through a thin area of mucous and binds to receptor sites on the olfactory nerve.

19

These receptor sites may be very specific, in that they are designed to detect particular odor molecules. We also know that some odor molecules respond better at some receptor sites than at others, which is part of the mechanism that allows us to discriminate between odors and identify odors that are present in our environment. Each of these receptors—and we have millions of them—will link with odor molecules that match them.

Once an odor molecule reaches a receptor site, the body's electrical signaling system begins operating. The odor molecule stimulates a long thin neuron nerve cell—known as the bipolar receptor cell—to fire. We can think of this as a stimulus- response, odor molecule-fire, mechanism. Now a representation of the odor molecule is transmitted up to the olfactory bulb at the top of the nose. The important point here is that the representation—or neural image or picture—of the odor changes. Through a complex mechanism, the original odor stimulus is intensified by a factor of one thousand. The intensified odor signal is projected through the olfactory bulb and reaches the main components of the brain. In other words, the system operates to take individual odor molecules and then intensifies them in such a way that the brain can respond to them.

Unlike the other senses, the olfactory gateway to the brain is direct. The cornea acts as a physical barrier between neurons in the visual processing system and stimuli in the outside world. Similarly, the eardrum acts as a barrier between the auditory processing apparatus and the sounds we hear. The nose provides no similar barrier.

From the Breath to the Brain

This journey of an odor signal through the olfactory bulb is necessary in order for the odor to reach structures throughout the limbic portion of the brain. Unlike our other senses, the receptors—or processors—for odor molecules are located in the emotional center of the brain. The limbic lobe of the brain, the seat of our emotional life, is located beneath the cerebral cortex, which is the intellectual, or cognitive, portion of the brain, and above the part of the brain stem that controls unconscious functions such as breathing and the workings of our internal organs.

The limbic lobe also activates the all-important hypothalamus, which is the control center for our drives and instincts, including our satiety center. It in turn sends messages to the pituitary, a tiny gland that releases hormones that regulate important functions of the body. The relationship between smell and appetite and weight loss has its roots in the pathway that odor molecules travel.

The limbic lobe of the brain is where we store emotional memories; it also controls our likes and dislikes, as well as anxiety, depression, joy, pleasure, anger, and so forth. This is why our sense of smell is such a powerful trigger for nostalgic reverie, based on nothing more than a whiff of an odor in the air. As we'll see in chapter 10, the nostalgic response, triggered by memories, may also have a role in food cravings and the sudden desire to eat.

The Brain Chemicals Do Their Part

Brain chemistry becomes involved in detecting and reacting to odors because a variety of neurotransmitters—chemicals in the brain—allow the nerve impulses to move from neuron to neuron in the olfactory bulb and on through the limbic lobe.

Neurotransmitters have many functions, including regulating mood and emotional well-being. Almost all the neurotransmitters found in the rest of the brain are found in the olfactory bulb, providing an additional indication that the link between our emotions and our sense of smell is no accident, but part of a careful design.

Your sense of smell is the only sensory system whose

stimuli are processed through the limbic portion of your brain before being processed by another critical part of the brain, the thalamus. The thalamus operates as a kind of relay station to and from the cerebral cortex. It plays an important role in sensation and signals the brain about environmental changes. With our sense of touch, for example, the cortex and the thalamus respond first, and then the limbic lobe becomes involved. You identify the texture of a fabric, and then you decide if you like or dislike it. Our vision works the same way. If I show you a picture of a cow or a horse or a tree, you process this through the eye and the thalamus and then through the area of the brain where vision is localized. At this point you interpret what you see; you decide that what you are looking at is a cow. After identifying the cow, the limbic system becomes involved, and now you decide if you like the cow. Obviously, these processes go on in imperceptible spans of time, and they go on constantly.

Smell works in the opposite way. Your sense of smell is designed to always react first, identify later. You decide if you like the smell before you project the signal off to the cortex to determine what the smell is. Without any logical thinking involved, you decide if you like or dislike an unfamiliar odor before you identify it. In other words, you have reactions to odors completely independent of your intellectual capacities. This explains how reactions to smell can be so irrational. There isn't anything rational about liking or disliking the smell of barbecued beef or a certain brand of floor wax or freshly cut roses. Yet you make these evaluations and judgments all the time.

Left Brain/Right Brain

Another way of understanding the emotional significance of smell is to look at the side of the brain in which smell is primarily processed. As you probably know, the left side of the brain controls such functions as logical thought, calculations, reading, and so forth. The right side of brain processes artistic endeavors, intuitive impulses, and other functions we associate with creativity.

Touch, sound, and vision are processed through the left side of the brain, the logical thinking control center. But smell is processed in the right side of the brain, the emotional and creative control center.

It's clear that these processes are outside our conscious control. We don't think about which side of the brain we're using when we listen to music, create a piece of sculpture, or chop vegetables for a stew. We don't turn off the emotional brain to do math any more than we turn off the thalamus once we have identified a cow. The processes are going on twenty-four hours a day, and we rarely give them much thought. Our senses work together and allow us to experience the world and function in our day-to-day lives. They are all part of a mechanism that ensures that we survive as individuals and as a species, and smell has a unique and important role in our preservation.

Our Survival May Be at Stake

Odors *need* to be processed in the emotional center of the brain precisely because it is so important for our survival. Early in human history, we needed to detect potential intruders invading our camp or territory, and our sense of smell helped us do that.

And it's important to remember that we react to odors we can't consciously detect. Odorous substances called pheromones are all around us, and we have evidence that they exist throughout the animal world, including that of the human family. Pheromones appear to have an important role in regulating many areas of human behavior, particularly our territorial drives and our sexuality. Unconsciously, pheromones allow us to sense the presence of other people or food sources. These invisible substances are also crucial for our survival.

Compared to the rest of the animal kingdom, we have a relatively weak sense of smell. The lowly cockroach has an ability to smell one hundred thousand times greater than our own. And, while the basic physiology of olfaction is markedly similar among mammals, through evolution the smell apparatus of humans has atrophied, meaning that it is smaller and less powerful than that of other primates.

I believe that our ancestors were aware of how important smell was in their lives, but in our modern era, vision has supplanted olfaction in what we think is most important. Overweight people say, for example, that they look at food and become hungry, when the truth is they usually detect the odor of food and have the conditioned response to either want to eat it if they like it or reject it if they don't. This response is not restricted to the obese, however. We all have it, but overweight individuals tend to link it with a problem, whereas normal-weight individuals don't.

Tears That Aren't from Sadness

An odor molecule is any substance that is designed to affect the olfactory nerve. However, what we describe as a smell is really a combination of an odor molecule and a stimulus to another nerve in the nose and face, the trigeminal nerve. This is an irritant nerve, stimulated when we cry, either from sadness or when we cut an onion, for example. This happens because stimulating the trigeminal nerve causes the eyes to burn. The trigeminal nerve is also involved when we sneeze in reaction to a substance that irritates the nasal passages. Again, this is a protective mechanism, allowing us to clear the irritant—purge it—before it can harm us.

We see the trigeminal nerve mechanism among people with no ability to smell at all. Logically, we would think that if we can't smell an onion, our eyes wouldn't sting, and we wouldn't cry. However, the trigeminal nerve knows when an odor is present and will respond whether we consciously detect the scent or not.

Sometimes we can treat people with olfactory loss by modifying their diets to include foods that stimulate the trigeminal nerve. Horseradish, chili peppers, and peppermint are examples of foods that will burn one's eyes. Our patients who eat these "irritating" foods don't notice improvement in their ability to smell, but they do have more sensations from eating.

If you've ever fainted and someone aroused you with smelling salts, you became alert again because the trigeminal nerve was stimulated, which in turn activated the part of the brain responsible for keeping us awake. But the process started with the odor that stimulated a particular nerve. Tear gas also activates this mechanism, which is why it forces people out of confined spaces and into the air, where the molecules are less dense. It may be experienced as burning eyes and difficult breathing, but the process started with an odor.

This Food Tastes Like Cardboard

If you pinch your nose and take a bite of an apple, you probably won't know it's an apple, and you might tell me that you just ate an onion. If you hold your nose and take a bite of the most expensive chocolate money can buy, you might as well have saved your money and eaten a piece of cardboard instead.

More than 90 percent of taste is actually smell, and taste is a misnomer in most cases anyway. We're physiologically equipped to distinguish four different categories of tastes: sweet, salty, sour, and bitter. Beyond that, we're really talking about flavor. Our experience of flavor results from the food's retronasal smell. The retronasal pathway goes from the back of the throat up to your nose. The odor molecules are released when we chew our food and make their way to the olfactory apparatus through this pathway. The retronasal mechanism is an alternate way to induce odorant substances to the olfactory bulb. We seldom think about the fact that we have this passageway, but recall a time in your life when you started coughing or choking while you were chewing some food or drinking a liquid. That chocolate cake or glass of milk came right out your nose! The retronasal mechanism also plays a role in triggering the signal that we've had enough to eat.

Women Have the Better Noses

While the basic mechanism of smell is the same for all human beings, differences in olfactory acuity cross gender and cultural lines. Women seem to believe they can smell better than their male companions—and they're usually right. A man often thinks that if he can't detect an odor, then the smell must not exist—the woman in his life must be imagining it. But men are often wrong when they insist that there is no smell of kerosene in the garage or gas in the kitchen, and they'd do well to listen to the women who are telling them otherwise.

Because nature doesn't seem to do anything from pure whimsy, women's superior olfactory acuity is probably another survival mechanism. A woman's ability to detect odors is highest when she is ovulating, leading us to believe that she can detect the pheromones of potential mates and be more receptive to mating at that time. And, since we know that female mammals must be able to identify their own young, it follows that women's better olfactory acuity is an additional evolutionary carryover, designed to help us survive. Many women also report increased appetite at the ovulatory phase of their cycles, and their increased olfactory ability during this time may help explain why this occurs. Women who are trying to lose weight may not appreciate that their premenstrual increased appetite is part of "nature's way," but knowledge may help them understand that this is not due to their weakness.

Subject to Change

As we age, our ability to detect and identify odors diminishes, which sometimes has a negative impact on nutritional status. Many older people don't eat enough because they forget to eat, in part because they don't detect the food odors around them. Likewise, our ability to smell may change because of trauma to the head, medications, and temporary or permanent diseases. Frankly, we're only beginning to understand the vast interplay between smell and our emotional, physical, and cultural lives.

We know that the satiety center in the hypothalamus exists for our protection. It's part of our complex mechanism of eating to live, but not to eat so much that we can't live. The role of our sense of smell in this survival game has been long underrated, and even dismissed, as not particularly important. But as our research is finding, the satiety center may contain an important secret for our modern problem of overabundance of food and consequent overeating. It appears that we can indeed fool nature—at least some of the time. That's what our research—and this book—is all about. Like most theories and helpful solutions, our odor-device program was the result of trial and error and a long journey.

The Great Chocolate Experiment

When we first began to correlate the role of smell in appetite control, we conducted a brief experiment, using medical students as our volunteers. At the beginning of each day, we gave the students a chocolate bar, which we thought of as a type of portable smell capsule. Whenever the students were hungry, they were supposed to pull out the chocolate and sniff it. We were trying to determine if having a whiff of the chocolate would activate, even momentarily, the satiety mechanism. Perhaps the chocolate would fool the satiety center, causing it to react as if candy had been eaten.

At the end of each day, we asked the students to report how their sensations of hunger fluctuated throughout the day and if the chocolate bar had helped keep them from impulsively eating any food available. We learned a few important things from these unsuspecting students. Like Pavlov's famous dogs, our students responded with perfect conditioning. They felt hungry, they sniffed the chocolate bars, they salivated, they ate the chocolate. Like so many of us, most of these students had a weakness for chocolate and couldn't resist—especially after taking a few sniffs. For some, the very presence of a chocolate bar was stimulus enough. On most days, the chocolate bars were consumed by early afternoon.

But, we also asked ourselves what would have happened if we had isolated the odor without providing the actual food. Would the satiety center have had a chance to work without the person actually consuming the food? In the absence of the immediate option to eat, would a sense of fullness or satisfaction be achieved through inhaling an odor alone? And, if so, would appetite be reduced enough to cause some weight loss?

Enter the Aroma Devices

To answer our questions, we organized a small, informal study. The device we used for the study was similar to a lipstick container that released an aroma. We asked our volunteers to sniff the odor any time they felt like doing so. We also asked them to tell us about their perceived fluctuations in appetite as well as any weight loss they experienced.

We were pleased when a significant number of people actually used the smell container regularly and also lost weight. Still, we couldn't consider the information definitive. People have a tendency to change their behavior during a study. For example, eating patterns could have subtly changed in ways that we couldn't accurately measure. Subjectively, the participants may have wanted the odor to work, and therefore, they ate less and lost a few pounds. We couldn't say for sure why they perceived reduced appetite, and therefore, we couldn't be sure that the weight loss wasn't due to the placebo effect.

Our next research project was a double-blind crossover study, using an aroma in a container and a placebo (the plastic odor of the container). Double-blind simply means that the researchers don't know which group is getting the placebo and which was getting the active substance. Therefore, when we tabulated the data, we didn't know which group was using the active odor. Crossover means that after a period of time—in this case, two weeks—the groups were switched, and those who initially received the odorized container were given the placebo for two weeks. Those who originally received the plastic odor were given the active odor.

All participants in this study were instructed not to change their eating patterns in any way, and they were asked not to change their exercise habits. The study subjects were instructed to use the odor whenever they wanted to, but especially when they felt hungry. While again our sample was small—105 people—the results were very encouraging. Weight loss on the placebo was too insignificant to be analyzed, while those who used the active odor lost an average of 1.5 pounds. Those with very good olfactory acuity lost more weight, almost 3 pounds. We could say that we were onto something that could help people fight evolution and perhaps, over time, lose significant amounts of weight.

Enter Green Apples, Peppermint, and Bananas

The results of our first studies encouraged us so much that we decided to launch a larger study and run it for a longer period of time. From our small project, we learned that people become tired of the same odor, and after a few days, it no longer has any appeal. It may even become an odor people will avoid. This is not surprising because most of us desire variety in our diets. We are attracted to different smells and tastes each day and eating the same foods again and again leads to feelings of deprivation. (This is an important cause of failure of most diets—the eating plans become boring, and the resulting sense of deprivation often leads to "cheating" just to add variety.)

In our research we also have found that people tend to prefer sweet smells, but our experience with chocolate tells us, in addition, that offering odors of very sweet, highly caloric food just might defeat our purpose. So, we chose the so-called neutral sweet smells that most study participants found pleasant but not overwhelming. Enter banana, green apple, and peppermint—and many willing people.

Putting a Human Face on the Research

Our study included 3,193 people, all of whom were given the three smells in small, canister-type tubes. This time our study participants were asked to sniff the odors three times in each nostril whenever they felt hungry. As in the first two studies, we gave them no special instructions about foods to eat or avoid and they were told not to change their exercise habits.

In order to gather as much scientific data as possible about the role of odors in weight loss, we tested each participant for the ability to smell. We used two olfactory tests, the same instruments we use to test patients who seek treatment for lack of olfactory acuity at our center. The participants also completed demographic questionnaires that documented age, race, religion, and so forth. Each was asked to take a psychological test as well as to complete two common standardized tests for depression (the Beck Depression Inventory and Zung Depression Scales). Each participant was also weighed at the beginning of the study and once a month thereafter.

Many of our participants came to Chicago from as far away as California, Florida—and even Canada. They agreed to fly to our center for their monthly weigh-ins and to have their progress assessed in other ways. Our participants represented many walks of life, as well as a variety of religions and ethnic backgrounds, and reported a wide range of life circumstances. The average age of our participant was forty-three and most (about 86 percent) were women.

It's important to note that most of our study subjects needed to lose significant amounts of weight—in many cases, more than 100 pounds. However, the typical volunteer was a woman about five feet five inches tall, weighing 217 pounds, and whose ideal weight was 129 pounds. She exercised about nine minutes a day, used alcohol moderately, and didn't smoke or use illegal substances. Many of our typical patients had gained and lost hundreds of pounds during their adult lives. It's fair to say that many were skeptical and, frankly, even angry about going through still one more attempt in their ongoing battle with obesity. But their willingness—skepticism notwithstanding—to try this at-that-time completely unknown method of appetite and weight control is a testimony to the deep desire many overweight people have to lead happier, healthier lives.

It seemed significant to us that so many of our study subjects were divorced, separated, or had never been married—only 13 percent were married and still living with their spouse. Although we don't like to talk openly about this in our society, obesity can contribute to many of life's problems. Some of our single subjects had withdrawn from seeking a life partner. They saw themselves in a painful cycle of gaining, losing, gaining, followed by increased isolation and emotional pain.

While our divorced and separated study subjects did not automatically link their weight problems to marital difficulties, they, too, saw themselves in a vicious circle. Sometimes they said that the stress of marital problems had contributed to their sense of despair over their obesity.

Indeed, the emotional toll of obesity in our thinness-worshiping society is profound. Throughout this book, you'll hear about some of the difficulties and the painful feelings experienced by overweight people. I relate this information and tell these stories not because I want to expose these individuals who so generously spoke to us but because I realize how many people in our society can relate to what our patients have told us. When more than half of a group of overweight people admit to hating themselves and are seriously dissatisfied with their lives, this indicates a serious problem that millions of people in our culture are dealing with every day. As a physician who is both a psychiatrist and a neurologist, I'm concerned about the emotional well-being of a large segment of our population. Even those study subjects who had learned to live well in spite of their obesity told us that painful, negative feelings about themselves were not infrequent.

Our Encouraging Results

In short, our larger and more lengthy study reported good news all around. Our results confirmed that odors can help people lose weight. Some people lost more than 100 pounds in the six-month study. In fact, the number one side effect of using the smell devices was *excess* weight loss! Some people lost so much weight that we had to drop them from the study—they actually became underweight. While the average weight loss of our participants was 5 pounds a month, we also found that those with better-than-average sense of smell lost weight more quickly than those on the low-end of normal. Our olfactory pretesting allowed us to confirm this.

Other important features of our study results will be discussed throughout this book (for a detailed report on the study, please see the appendix). You'll learn about the habits of those who had the most rapid weight loss and about the supplementary activities you can do to enhance an odor-based program. But, the most important finding was our demonstration that using active odors can indeed help you lose weight. Furthermore, it doesn't seem to matter if you have 20 pounds to lose or 220, the results are the same. Sure, it will take more than a few weeks to lose 50 pounds or more, but given the high failure rate of diets, this shouldn't discourage you. In fact, you might find yourself at last fulfilling your long-standing dream of achieving—and not just temporarily—a normal weight.

An Important Additional Benefit

When I first began to study the relationship between the satiety mechanism and smell, I believed that the primary reason, perhaps even the sole reason, the smell devices work had to do with fooling the brain. This does seem to be true, but another important benefit of using the smell canister has become clear to us.

Just as we have learned to respond to the smell of certain foods by feeling hungry and wanting to eat, we can, in a very real sense, "unlearn" or deprogram ourselves. For many people the smell of any food triggered hunger. Smell a doughnut, salivate; smell a pizza, and the stomach growls. Actually, most of us experience this much of the time; but in the overweight person, this conditioned, or learned, response can be quite powerful.

It's exciting to realize that people can recondition themselves to smell an odor and *not* respond with hunger. In the absence of a food associated with the smell, hunger disappeared, the desire to eat subsided, and a pattern was broken. In many cases, this was a long-standing pattern that was broken during the six-month study.

Thirty-year-old Sherry told us, "It was like a reflex response—smell, see, eat. Now I grab the smell canister, and it's as if I learned a new habit." The presence of a new habit is exactly the benefit that we couldn't have foreseen with any certainty. Smell can be used as an intrinsic part of learning to live—and eat—in an entirely new way.

The Future Is Now

Had we known decades ago about the relationship among the sense of smell, odors, and weight and appetite control, we might have avoided the epidemic of obesity that currently afflicts so many of us. But we didn't have this information until recently, and the past is the past. The study of olfaction and its role in many areas of human life is a revolution in itself. For example, you now have a variety of these smell devices available to you; soon they will become commonplace. Perhaps they will eventually be marketed to help people stop smoking, to improve concentration, or for any number of reasons. We're already learning that a variety of smells affect the brain in different ways.

However, for your purposes, you can use these devices to help you maximize your often-forgotten sense of smell. You can use a unique form of aromatherapy to fool nature's satiety mechanism and to learn new habits. Unlike our study participants who were limited to three smells, you can use the wide variety of smells available to you in many forms. For example, as you'll learn in chapter 7, you may choose to add scents to your home that induce a calm, relaxed mood. Indeed, many people eat more when they are nervous, and you might have noticed this correlation on your own.

So far, we've talked about the reasons for rampant obesity in our modern society. We've also discussed the satiety center in the brain and have some preliminary information about how it works and the way smell can be used to fool it. In the next chapters, you'll see how you can use food and its smells to start a safe program of appetite and weight control. You'll learn tips about using everyday aromas and smell devices in a practical—and possible—way. No diets, no forbidden foods. And, most certainly, this system doesn't try to make food unpleasant or unappealing. You'll enjoy your meals as you always have, but like our study participants, you'll find that you're eating less. As you begin to lose weight and feel better about your health and well-being, you'll also gain some insights into the many reasons you may have used food to cope with stress and anxiety. You aren't so different from other people, and you'll learn how often most of us reach for food to comfort us, even when we aren't consciously aware of being anxious or frustrated.

Many people have now learned how to use odors at home, at the office, and in many other settings. This same information is now available to you, and you'll be surprised how easy it is to bring these odors into your day-to-day life.

3 Sniff Away—
Using the Odors

When we started our study, we told participants to use the odor devices whenever and wherever they felt hungry, or during those times when they believed they would be especially tempted by food. Our instructions were to inhale three times in each nostril whenever they used the device. This system brought about the best results for our participants.

These guidelines worked well, and they're the same ones I'm recommending to you. We found that people tended to adapt them to their daily routines quite easily. The most important thing to remember is that *smell devices work best when they are used frequently.* Some participants took more than three hundred sniffs a day. The other key to success is to be sure that you have the device with you. Carry it in your pocket, handbag, briefcase, and so forth. Keep devices in your car, on your nightstand, in the bathroom, and by all means, in the kitchen.

One woman complained that she didn't think the device was working because she went to a restaurant and ate more than she'd planned. I asked her if she'd used the device prior to her meal. As it turned out, she forgot to bring it with her, and then she wondered why the sniffing she'd done earlier in the day hadn't "carried over," so to speak. It doesn't work that way. The devices can't work if you don't use them when you need them, at the time you will be facing food. Your morning's sniffs aren't going to help you at dinner. As you begin to use the odors, you'll understand what I mean. Let's look at some typical patients and see how they adjusted to the odors.

Waking Up with the Odors

We can call Barbara a typical study participant. She needed to lose about 70 pounds, the same number of pounds she'd lost about two years before entering our study. She'd rebounded and now was looking for another way to lose the weight and keep it off—she couldn't face another diet.

Barbara was skeptical, as many of our study subjects were. She had never tried to lose weight without a list of foods she could eat and another list of foods to avoid. She had intense food cravings, mostly for sweets and chocolate. But, discouraged though she was, she took the three inhalers home and vowed to use them. When the alarm clock went off the next morning, she reached for the inhaler, did the three sniffs in each nostril and went about her morning routine. She inhaled again as she started preparing her breakfast, and much to her surprise, she left half the bowl of cereal she'd fixed and ate only half a piece of toast. She felt full and stopped eating.

By mid-morning she was feeling a bit hungry, but she hadn't yet used the inhaler in her office. When a coworker brought in a bag of doughnuts for the coffee break snack, she remembered that she had the inhaler in her purse. As she put it, "I made a beeline for the restroom and sniffed six times. I don't know why, it changed something. I wasn't hungry for the doughnut—and I always want sweets in any form. I accepted the doughnut, took two bites, and then quickly threw the rest away. No one noticed what I'd done."

We asked Barbara why she had accepted the doughnut in the first place, considering that she hadn't felt hungry. "It was just habit," she said, "and I didn't want to call attention to myself in the office. If I'd turned the doughnut down, people would have started talking about 'Barbara's new diet,' and I didn't want that to happen. If you announce you're on a diet, people start watching what you eat. Even worse, they start commenting on it."

Barbara makes a good point. Some of our study participants kept quiet about the odor devices for the same reason Barbara chose to. She didn't want to call attention to herself, so she used the inhaler in the restroom—at least at first. By the time lunch hour arrived, Barbara had used the odor device in the ladies' room of the restaurant; she ordered a regular lunch and ate half of it. She was eating alone that day and read a magazine while she ate. This was typical for her, so she hadn't changed her routine at all.

Barbara worked in a very food-oriented office, not unlike millions of workplaces across the country (and we wonder why it's so difficult to stick to diets!). Almost every morning and afternoon, someone went out for snacks. Determined to "keep her own counsel," she again accepted a muffin from the bakery in her building, ate a few bites, and threw the rest away. Barbara's work involves being on the telephone, often handling customer service issues for much of the day. Her office is a social place, where these morning and afternoon food excursions are a daily occurrence. She knew she would have to contend with the food being placed in front of her, but she also stayed determined not to let her "diet" become the talk of the office.

After work, Barbara met a friend for an early dinner. Barbara decided to order a full meal, even though she felt odd about having a baked potato and dinner rolls with butter, which are not typical "diet" fare. As soon as she ordered, she used the odor device in the restroom; afterward, she left food on her plate. After using the inhaler in the ladies room again later, she ate less than half of the dessert she'd ordered.

At the end of the evening, just before bed, Barbara had

a strong craving for sweets—the kind of craving that, in the past, had driven her to the nearest convenience store. This time she took out the inhaler and sniffed, not three times, but about a dozen times over the next few minutes. "The craving subsided," she said, "and I was able to get ready for bed without feeling cheated. Once a craving starts, it's difficult to stop thinking about it, but the inhaler helped. It was so different that I began to think about the device instead of food."

Barbara's first day on the odor plan was fairly typical, in that she ate some of everything, but didn't finish everything on her plate. She was able to go along with her coworkers during their snack time and enjoy an evening meal with a friend. "Except for eating less," Barbara said, "my routine hadn't changed."

One of the advantages of the odor devices is that it isn't disruptive and doesn't require special food preparation and the tedious measuring and weighing that so many dieters complain about. As the week went on, Barbara tried to follow our advice and not focus on weight loss but, rather, focus on using the device. This is very difficult, of course. We understood that our participants would be tempted to weigh themselves every day or every few days. We certainly didn't keep them from doing that, but we assured them that the once-a-month weigh-in would be sufficient.

Barbara did weigh herself at the end of the week and she'd lost three pounds. She got a bit overconfident, and during the second week, she began to forget to use the odor device before her meals and snacks. Her weight loss was only one pound that week, which was disappointing to her. She stepped up the use of the inhaler during the third and fourth weeks, stopped weighing herself, and was again eating significantly less food. Her total weight loss during the first month was 7.5 pounds—a very good and healthy start.

The best part for Barbara was that it was such painless weight loss. She was still eating a couple of bites of the sweets with her coworkers and she never mentioned what she was doing. In fact, Barbara waited until she'd lost about 25 pounds before she confided in a few friends. They were astonished by how she'd done it, mainly because they hadn't noticed any change in her eating habits. Some wanted to know about the study and called for information. Word of mouth started to spread through Barbara's circle of friends and acquaintances. In fact, one of her friends signed up for our study, and now he, too, has lost weight.

Why All the Snacks—Why No Food Plan

The very word "diet" strikes fear in the hearts of people who have gained and lost weight over a lifetime. The word itself implies deprivation, sacrifice, hunger, and so forth. When we decided to experiment with odors, we wanted to see if scents would affect eating behavior and if weight could be lost without other lifestyle changes. If we had added a food plan or mandated exercise, we would have confused the results by having too many variables. Our results certainly showed that odors alone can promote weight loss.

I believe that many of our study subjects would benefit from better diets, and most would certainly feel better if they exercised more. But, deprivation is probably worse for people than a few bites of a doughnut in the morning or a half a chocolate chip cookie in the afternoon.

Barbara was able to live normally *and lose weight*. Nothing can beat that combination. Most people can't stay on diets indefinitely, and even if they do, they must cope, from the first day, with changing their routines. No one in her office had a clue that Barbara was using scent devices in the restroom or alone in her home. She told people about her new weight loss plan when she was ready.

Did Barbara feel uncomfortable about "sneaking" around with her inhaler? Not at all. She had worked in the same office for more than ten years. Her coworkers had seen her gain and lose hundreds of pounds—25 pounds one year, 35 the next, right up to 70 pounds on one commercial diet. Barbara had a closet filled with clothes from size ten all the way up. She had been in the habit of announcing each new diet. On some of them, she brought prepared food to heat in the microwave; for others, she brought special food to the office that she'd weighed and measured at home. Naturally, people asked about her diet, how it was going, and how much weight she'd lost. "I'd made the mistake of talking too much before," she said, "and I wasn't going to let that happen again. During one Christmas party, a coworker actually took a plate of food away from me." Apparently, thinking that he was being helpful, her coworker said, "Now, Barbara, you don't really want to blow you diet. Let me get rid of this." He proceeded to dump the food in the trash. Later that night, Barbara binged on sweets—she felt like a child who'd been chastised for doing something wrong. "It was only wrong," she said, "because I had told everybody that I was on a diet—no one else was under that kind of scrutiny."

As the months went by, Barbara began using the inhaler more often. In fact, she got through the next holiday season not by depriving herself of food but, as she said, "by sniffing my way through parties." Even during the big family dinners, she was able to put her fork down after tasting a few bites of everything. She never felt deprived, and her weight loss continued. "Some evenings, I used the inhaler a dozen times or more," she said. "I had a few rocky times, but the odors came to the rescue."

It took Barbara less than a year to lose 70 pounds. As she got closer to her goal weight and she could see that this was not just another diet scheme, she was able to be more open to suggestions about changing her diet and increasing exercise. Feeling better, emotionally and physically, Barbara could address the lifelong issues of maintaining a normal weight.

It's Not Necessary to Go It Alone

Barbara had valid reasons for keeping news of her diet to herself. Other people, however, are better off with a support system of some kind. These individuals feel good when people encourage them to lose weight, comment on their changing appearance, and so forth. This decision is entirely up to you.

Cindy and Alice, two members of our program, illustrate the value of having a "smell buddy," something we recommend to couples or friends who start the odor program together. Cindy and Alice became acquainted when they were in the same commercial diet program, four years before they entered our study. The women signed up together and traveled for their monthly weigh-ins and checkups as a team. They worked at opposite ends of their city, but they called each other every morning during the first month of the program to offer each other mutual support. Later they had less need for a morning check-in, even though they stayed in contact because they had become close friends.

Cindy had about 110 pounds to lose, Alice about 85 pounds. Both were raising children alone and had been through some very difficult times. Because of the stress in their lives, neither felt up to another diet, but both very much wanted to lose weight. Cindy had been told that the joint problems she was experiencing were a direct result of her obesity; Alice had once liked to play tennis and volley-ball, but she had given both up because she was embarrassed by the way she looked.

Alice was not the only person who talked about the shame she felt at the gym or even out walking. Having once been active, she found it very difficult to isolate herself in her home, but believed she had no other choice. It would be easy for me to say, "That's nonsense. You should do whatever exercise you can and to heck with what other people think." My words, however, would fall on deaf ears.

Besides, that's what other people tell the Alices of the world, and what good has it done? In our society, one that worships at the door of thinness while simultaneously exalting food, overweight people are subject to these cruel mixed messages all the time. Telling them not to care is like telling them not to breathe.

Cindy hadn't even considered exercising, except for an occasional walk. Her knees and ankles were stiff and sore, and exercise was torture. She also felt as Alice did, that going to a gym was too humiliating and they'd had enough humiliation to last a lifetime. Since exercise wasn't part of our research protocol—although I believe strongly in it both for losing and maintaining weight—it wasn't an issue for us whether they exercised or not. What concerned me more was that they had allowed obesity to drive them into isolation and that they felt almost obligated to hide from others. It was Alice who told us, "Overweight women are pariahs in this country."

Cindy pointed out that isolation is easier than it would seem: "When you're raising two kids alone, there's so much to do that going to work and staying home the rest of the time isn't difficult. Finding time to do things? Now that's work."

Because they were both so busy, the idea of being smell buddies appealed to them. They could talk first thing in the morning while packing their children's lunches, check in during lunch hour, and again at night if they needed to. Their sign-off was "keep sniffing!" Once, when Alice was in a supermarket buying groceries for her kids, she saw one of her "binge" foods and picked it up. Then she remembered that she could call Cindy and talk to her, and that thought helped her put the food down. As soon as she left the store, she called her smell buddy and told her what had happened. Just having someone to talk to was a relief. At least Cindy understood why she'd had the close call with food.

Alice and Cindy were able to exchange tips about using

the smell devices and that also helped them enjoy the novelty of this way of losing weight. After a week or two, both commented that using the inhaler instead of eating so much food with each meal turned out not to be so very difficult after all. Both women realized within the first month that the more they sniffed the less they ate. This is the idea, of course, but people don't believe it until they try it for themselves.

As they compared notes, both found that sniffing the inhaler before, during, and after a meal worked best. Cindy pointed out that while she could leave food on her plate, she would feel like eating within minutes of clearing the table. Sniffing the odors again relieved the urge to eat. I believe she was using the inhaler to break a habit. She wasn't hungry after her dinner—she was frustrated, and the stress of the day caught up with her. Eating was a way to manage, or modulate, her stress. Many people do this, of course, even the very slim. Cindy noticed it because having the odor device available to her gave her something else to do that was a reasonable substitute for eating. She was able to connect her urge to eat with wanting comfort or an emotional fortification to get through the rest of her evening chores. Alice reminded Cindy about the importance of not depriving herself of regular meals. This was an important function of the smell buddy concept. Cindy might have quickly turned this program into a deprivation diet had not Alice encouraged her to eat.

The two women also compared notes about how often they sniffed the three different inhalers, and both confirmed that it's better to switch the odors every day. Becoming bored with a smell reduces its effectiveness. In fact, people who used only the banana scent because they especially liked that odor eventually got so tired of the smell that they stopped using the devices. People often stop dieting because they become so sick of the food they're allowed to eat that they can't face it. Variety is the spice of life—and it's certainly true of food and odors. As time goes on, more and more scents will be available, so variety shouldn't be an issue over the long run.

If you decide to use the odors to lose weight, remember that you need food to live. Don't immediately turn this program into a diet. And remember: eating three small meals and two snacks is much better than sniffing all day and then eating an oversized dinner and munching all evening. Many dieters have tried to eat almost nothing during the day so that they can enjoy a big dinner. This was most common during the decades of calorie counting. The typical woman dieter was "allowed" about one thousand calories, so if she was going out to dinner or to a special party or celebration, she attempted to "save" her precious allotment. However, this plan doesn't work because the inevitable result is over-eating. In addition, a person trying this often ends up feeling weak and empty all day and then overstuffed at night. *Sniffing the odors isn't a substitute for a meal; rather, the odors are an adjunct to meals.*

Cindy and Alice lost weight rapidly. They used the odor devices regularly and often—up to two hundred fifty sniffs a day. Like most participants, they tried to avoid sniffing in front of other people—except each other. Both used them in the car on the way to work, in restrooms, and then again at home. One evening, when they hired a baby-sitter and went to a movie together, they took many sniffs from the inhaler before finding their seats and sniffed during the movie in the darkened theater. They did this because the odor of the buttered popcorn was very tempting. At one time, they would have avoided movie theaters and felt deprived of both food and entertainment. Now they were able to enjoy an evening out.

After six months in the study, both women were buying new clothes in much smaller sizes. Better yet, they had begun to exercise, and Alice had joined a tennis club. Cindy was able to walk for up to an hour, and her joint pain was considerably reduced. And even better, both learned a lot about themselves and why they had engaged in so much overeating.

Alice and Cindy will eventually curtail their use of the odor device; neither will continue sniffing two hundred times a day or more. They won't need to. The break from overeating has allowed them to form new habits, and the odor device will always be there if they need it. These two women helped each other as only true friends can. Our foundation gave them the guidelines, and we monitored their progress, but their bond was what helped them more than any other single factor.

Partners, Not Competitors

In our study, we also had husband and wife smell buddies, a system that can work well in some cases. Since men tend to lose weight faster than women, however, it is important not to engage in a competition over who can drop pounds more quickly, and it is not a good idea to monitor each other's food intake.

Spouses are not the only people vulnerable to this subtle pressure that ends up being a rivalry—even a friendly one. Mothers and daughters can also develop a competitive attitude, which isn't good for their relationship, especially when it comes to weight loss. Again, it's not the smell buddy's job to monitor what the other person eats. Sharing tips for using odors and offering support is a positive role that avoids burdening either person with criticism or too much advice. (If there's one thing most seasoned dieters are sick of, it's well-meaning advice—so much of it turns out to be irrelevant in their cases, not to mention wrong. Remember that at one time, overweight women were advised to smoke cigarettes to control their appetites—"Reach for a Lucky instead of a sweet," was an actual advertising slogan. We know now how dangerous that advice turned out to be.)

Cindy and Alice discussed potential problems before they began calling each other. They agreed to some ground rules, one of which was that they wouldn't discuss specific foods unless it was important for some reason. Food items or categories of food turned out to be significant only when they felt a bit discouraged and were tempted to buy and consume products that were associated with comfort. For both Cindy and Alice, certain foods had become handy and easy substitutes for companionship. Their mutual support helped them use the program effectively, get through some hard times and, most important, offer each other hope.

Addiction or Habit?

Brent was concerned that he'd become addicted to sniffing the odors. "I've been addicted to other things in my life, and now I'm afraid of becoming hooked on these inhalers. Is there any danger of that?"

Brent's question wasn't unusual. He had a history of alcoholism and had been a heavy smoker as well. He had been free of alcohol for almost twelve years, however, and had quit smoking about six years before we met him. His battle with smoking was harder than with alcohol, perhaps because nicotine is so addictive, but also because drinking had adversely influenced his behavior, making his motivation to quit using alcohol strong. He would have lost both his job and his family had he not addressed his illness and the problems it had brought into his life.

Addiction is a word we use rather loosely nowadays; it is important to distinguish addiction from habit. People do indeed become physically addicted to many types of pre-scription and recreational drugs and, of course, to alcohol. Gambling is a behavioral addiction, and support groups have formed in which people help each other recover and normalize their lives. Overeaters Anonymous was formed to help people break abusive and even addictive behavior around food. In general, antisocial and self-destructive behavior are associated with addictions. As we all know, people addicted to alcohol can bring themselves and their families to ruin, as can gambling addicts, who might even be driven to steal in order to keep their habit going. (This is not speculation; statistics on youthful offenders have demonstrated this again and again.) Smoking is a powerful addiction and often has devastating consequences for one's health. While nonsmokers might not like to be around cigarette smoke, however, we wouldn't say that smokers are antisocial or driven to immoral behavior. It's an addiction where the health hazards are great, and the primary victim is the user.

Unfortunately, in recent years we've tended to talk about habitual behavior as addiction. Therefore, if people tend to habitually pick the wrong partners, we say they're addicted to bad relationships. Or, if a person enjoys running marathons or jogs a certain number of miles each day, we say he or she is addicted to exercise. It's true that people who exercise regularly miss it terribly when their routine is disrupted. They may even be a bit uncomfortable because they are in the habit of jogging every day, and it seems like something is missing. True exercise addiction is very rare, however, and not something most people need to concern themselves with in the least.

Most people have routines and habits. It's been said that we're all creatures of habit. I know people who eat the same breakfast at the same time every day of their lives, and I would never say they were addicted to that breakfast food. They are in the habit of eating certain foods, and their habit hurts no one, including themselves.

Using the odors on a regular basis becomes habitual. People who find them helpful just naturally start to remember to bring them along when they leave the house—we instruct them to do so. Most of our study subjects carried the inhalers around the house, and when food thoughts started intruding, they reached for the device and were then able to put their mental focus elsewhere. This is a habit— I don't think it's an addiction. Even if the people begin to feel uncomfortable or a bit nervous because they forget the device, so what? What is better, to be unhappy at an unhealthy weight or to have a harmless habit of using odors to curb appetite, reduce weight, reverse physical damage, and lower risk factors for many illnesses?

One of our participants had her purse stolen a few weeks after she started our program, and her odor device was taken along with her purse. We received a frantic call to send her another device right away; she felt lost without it. She felt lost for the simple reason that she was losing weight and didn't want to break her momentum for even one day. She'd formed the habit of sniffing the odor before and after each meal, and often in between meals, especially in the evening. She felt more freedom, not less, because she was released from a kind of bondage—she'd come to believe that food was an enemy that was holding her captive. The odor device was a method to change her behavior in a positive way. She'd never felt better in her adult life. She'd stopped overeating, and her excess pounds were coming off. Of course we sent her another inhaler immediately. We certainly didn't worry about her "habit." For the time being, she was "hooked" on reaching a healthful weight.

In order for our program to work, you need to form the habit of using the inhaler on a regular basis. A hit-and-miss approach is ineffective. We aren't encouraging addiction. We're encouraging you to break the old habit of eating more food than your body needs and instituting the habit of using odors to help you lose and maintain a weight that is right for you.

Brent's family was understandably concerned about any behavior that could seem like a harmful addiction. Once he was reassured that using odors was nothing more than forming a habit, just like the habit he'd developed of walking an hour four times a week, he felt better. When he explained to his family the difference between habits and destructive addictions, they all felt much better. He also realized that eventually his new way of eating would become a habit and that he was free to use the odors when he needed them and curtail his use if he maintained his weight over a long period of time.

If you have suffered from obesity and know the pain of the yo-yo syndrome, I would make using the odors your first priority. I would not worry about forming a habit that you can't break. The people who lost the most weight on our program are those who used the devices liberally. They sniffed anytime, anywhere. To them, it was the best possible habit they could have imagined.

Throughout this book, we'll discuss all the possible reasons that the odor devices work so well. The reasons include changes in brain chemistry, breaking social conditioning, and a host of other factors. But the success of using odors for weight loss can also be attributed to breaking one habit and forming another. People eat for many reasons, and using the odor devices offers a chance to substitute a helpful scent for an unneeded second helping. The substitute also provides a break in a pattern—and old habit—and allows individuals to examine the reasons they crave certain foods or automatically fill their stomachs with too much food.

Write It All Down

Food diaries or progress journals were not a part of our research protocol, but participants who did some journal writing found it very helpful. Most avoided the strict food diary format, however. They concentrated instead on how they felt during the program and didn't associate the writing with a "diet." In some cases, keeping a journal was helpful in giving participants greater insight into why they had the urge to eat.

Sarah had been overweight as a child, and food had become the focus of her adult life, too. She literally lived to eat. Before she entered our program, she had established a kind of informal agenda for her life. She went to work at a job that was not very demanding, and when she came home, she ate—and ate and ate. As she ate, she thought about losing weight and tried to figure out which new diet she would start. She had never stayed on a diet more than a week— the feelings of deprivation were too much for her to handle.

Sarah heard about our program and decided to try it. She had also entered therapy and was working on many personal issues, too. Her journal was a vehicle for exploring her patterns, and she wrote in it every evening—usually after using the odor inhaler for the last time that day. The journal helped her understand the emotional cycle that she'd been caught in for years. The odor device helped her start a new cycle, and her journal writing helped her therapy proceed as well. Sarah lost weight quite quickly, and she recorded her feelings about the weight loss in her journal. She had a record to look back on from time to time, and this gave her great strength.

Many people in our study told us that they had once thought that there were just two ways to eat. They either ate everything in sight and felt stuffed and even ill, or they were on a diet. The idea of eating smaller amounts of whatever they felt like eating that day was almost foreign to them. This is where using the odor devices combined with keeping a journal helped so many. Sarah particularly became fascinated with what she called "normal living and normal eating." Sarah told us about her plans to find a job that made better use of her college degree, something she hadn't been motivated to do before, mainly because, as she put it,

"I didn't want anything to interfere with my eating—even a demanding, but fulfilling job. Now I know I can live a normal life, including building a great career."

Another way a journal can be helpful is if it becomes a substitute for continuing to eat. Mike usually ate lunch with various people in his office. Once he started using the inhaler, however, he excused himself and found a place to be alone in order to write down whatever came to mind. He told his colleagues that he was working on a writing project and didn't mean to be antisocial; he needed the extra time for his project. No one questioned him, and he was free to leave the table while others were still eating.

I encourage you to keep a journal and fill it with anything and everything you want to. Don't feel you must use it as a food diary—record what you're eating only if that makes you feel better. Some people like to write about their progress; other people just write what they're thinking about that day. Choose your own way.

Lighten Up

One day we received an unusual phone call at our office. One of our study participants is a secretary who used the odor device quite a bit and lost weight rapidly. In fact, she put her head under her desk frequently in order to do her sniffing. She tried to be surreptitious and thought her behavior had gone unnoticed. But her boss spotted her and became suspicious. He thought she had taken to using drugs and was even ingesting them in the office under her desk. And, he thought, don't drug users lose weight? Finally, he asked her about this disturbing behavior, and when she told him she was using an odor inhaler to lose weight, he thought she must be joking, crazy, or lying.

She urged him to call our office, and when we explained—verified, really—what she was doing, he was amazed. Relieved and wanting to learn more, we told him about our theory and the study we designed. He asked how soon he could come in and sign up!

I predict that one day in the not-too-distant future, people will be talking about their odor inhalers rather than their diets. Instead of comparing calorie charts, people will be talking about the latest new odor on the market. If this all seems amusing, I'm glad. We're studying the science of odors in many areas of life, including weight loss. Science is serious business—no doubt about it. But applying science doesn't have to be dreary or boring—it can even be funny. Many of our patients have learned to laugh over their "smell adventures."

Are There Any People Who Shouldn't Use the Inhalers?

Fortunately, the smell devices are safe for almost everyone. But there are exceptions. If you have asthma, you can still use your nose for weight loss, but it isn't advisable for you to sniff the devices. In the next chapter, I describe ways to use your sense of smell without the odor devices, and while it might not be as easy to lose weight, an asthma attack obviously is worse.

People who suffer from migraine headaches need to use the devices with great care, if at all. Some might find that particular odors trigger a headache. Individuals are generally aware of this, however, and will be able to determine whether using the inhaler is a good idea.

I also do not want to see people of normal weight using inhalers to become thinner than they should be. Remember, the number one side effect of our study was too much weight loss! We are not promoting extreme thinness, and the waiflike models of our day are very bad role models for young women. If you are normal weight and have the urge to lose pounds in order to fit an unrealistic image, I'd prefer that you seek counseling to examine the reasons you want to be thinner.

It's So Easy to Get Started

All you need to begin this program are odor inhalers. It doesn't matter if you're in a study or not, this program can work for you. Some simple guidelines follow.

- Sniff the inhalers as many times a day as you like. Each time you use the device, inhale three times in each nostril. The whole process takes less than a minute. In our study, the more often people used the device, the more weight they lost.

- Take the odor device with you wherever you go—literally. Keep one in your pocket, in the car, near your bed, on the bathroom sink counter, most certainly in the kitchen, and in the living room, too. Make sure you have one available where you work. Our study subjects worked in stores, factories, offices, at outdoor construction sites, and in home-based businesses. If you leave town, make sure you have a supply with you. You can lose weight even on vacation. And use them at parties and holiday dinners—if you do, you might be the only person who doesn't leave the table feeling stuffed and sleepy.

- Vary the odors. We get tired of the same food because we are tired of the same smells. If you become tired of a smell, the very thought of it might make you ill or, more typically, bore you so that you won't use the inhaler as much.

- If a smell buddy will help you, find one. Just be sure that you and your buddy are offering mutual support and do not become competitive. It doesn't matter who loses faster. A sense of well-being is the most important benefit of this program.

- If you prefer to protect your privacy, you aren't obligated to tell anyone what you're doing. Many of our participants used the odors in the privacy of their homes and in restrooms at their places of work. Barbara was concerned that other people would monitor what she was eating, so she was very wise to keep her new program to herself. Soon enough there will be a time and place to talk to other people about odors and weight loss.

- Keep a journal if you want to. As I've said, many patients find it helpful. If it seems burdensome to you, don't do it. It's not mandatory. Using the odor devices is the only requirement.

- Don't be concerned with a food plan or restrictions on your diet just now. You may be a "seasoned" dieter. You know the ropes, so to speak, and can recite the number of calories in every food from pasta to mangoes. You probably know how many fat grams are in four ounces of skinless chicken and a fast food burger. Some of our participants were so accustomed to dieting that they assumed they *should* change the foods they ate. I'd much rather have people sniffing away pounds by consuming less of what they normally eat than by thinking in terms of calories and measuring cups of vegetables and trying to tell the difference between a medium-size apple and a large one. As you progress, you can think about more healthful eating, but you will never have to feel deprived.

This is all you need to get started. Now you know why losing weight is so difficult and how and why odors might be able to help. In the next chapter, I'll deepen your understanding of how odors can fool the brain and give you some additional tips for losing weight that involve your sense of smell but do not require using the odor device.

4 *Sniffing without the Device*

When we decided to use odors to promote weight loss, we were taking advantage of a built-in mechanism that exists to protect us and ensure our survival. A food odor is projected up to the satiety center, which then triggers the satiety mechanism. You don't need an odor device to see this for yourself. If you cook aromatic spaghetti sauce in your kitchen all day long, chances are you won't feel like eating very much of it by the time it's done—even if you've been looking forward to it all day.

The way the satiety center works also shows us that it can, so to speak, be fooled. That's the purpose of the smell devices. In other words, this center can behave—or react—as if you have eaten when you haven't. Some people shouldn't use the smell devices because they have asthma or are subject to migraine headaches, making the use of odor inhalers inappropriate in most cases. However, these individuals may still benefit from using the sense of smell to fool the satiety center. In addition, those who use odor inhalers can augment them by learning to use the odors that naturally occur in our food.

Obesity Is Complex, No Solution Is Simple

The information I'm presenting in this chapter is for any one who would like to lose some weight. But you must understand that the issue of appetite, weight, and weight loss is very complex. In other words, people with minor weight problems might see some results from a simple device such as a flavored mouth spray or by cooking aromatic food and sniffing the odors before they eat. However, for those with serious weight problems, these methods, including our own smell device, should be used as *one* remedy among many. Our research protocol was carefully designed, and each person was monitored throughout the study. As I've said, we didn't design a food plan or an exercise program. But research is not the same as "real life." As a physician, I'm concerned that you deal with a weight problem in a safe, effective way. What we call morbid obesity, meaning that excess weight seriously threatens health, should be treated medically. In many cases, medical treatment is augmented with psychological help.

The tips that follow are safe for everyone, and if you want to lose a small amount of weight (5–15 pounds), these small but significant ideas may help you. If you want to lose larger amounts of weight, these ideas represent tools you can use along with the smell devices, a food plan you may be following, an exercise program (more on exercise in chapter 8), and medical supervision.

In essence, these ideas help you consciously use your sense of smell—one of your most valuable resources for weight control—to fool the satiety center in the brain. Again, the goal is to feel satisfied without eating as much food as you normally would.

Sniffing before the First Bite

Smell your food before you eat it. Let the odor molecules travel up your nose, stimulating the olfactory nerve. The odor projects through the olfactory bulb and on to the hypothalamus, the master gland of the brain. Hence, you begin stimulating the satiety center before you begin eating. Patients I've worked with have commented that this often helps them eat a bit less at every meal. The principle here is the same, of course, as that associated with the artificial smell device.

You might notice that some people seem to enthusiastically sniff their food without thinking about it very much. A friend of mine is often a bit embarrassed when he is "caught" with his nose in the food platters and serving bowls. My friend is very thin, and this may not be entirely accidental. You might observe too, that people who smell cooking odors with great gusto may be the slimmer among us, or at least they are not battling a chronic weight problem.

Some people sniff everything before they eat it, from the strawberry jam they're spreading on their toast to the platter of chicken curry in the restaurant where they're sharing dinner with friends. The tendency to sniff food is a protective one, of course. Food odors are pleasurable for the most part, but bad food smells alert us to food that has gone bad. This is another example of how important our sense of smell is—our survival sometimes depends on it. Nowadays, however, smelling food before we eat it is probably habitual, and it's a habit worth developing.

Chew and Chew Again

Take only small bites of food and chew each bite well. Some of you, like our patients, might be thinking, "Oh, that again." Overweight people are often told to chew their food very well. It's usually advice given in an effort to slow them down. But there is another rationale for this valuable tip. The natural odors of food are released when you chew each bite well. Small amounts of well-chewed food allow the smell to affect the hypothalamus and possibly fool it into believing that more food has been ingested than is actually the case. The odor molecules reach the olfactory bulb through the retronasal passage at the back of the throat.

Chewing food well also slows the pace of eating, which is an additional benefit. Much has been written about the American way of gulping down food as if we've pulled into a gas station and are "refueling." We eat breakfast on the run, sometimes standing up in the kitchen or even while driving. Then we might gulp our lunch in ten minutes at our desks or eat quickly at a restaurant, usually fighting the clock. Then we pick up the kids from school and rush home, perhaps to cook, but sometimes to pack everyone in the car again to rush to the drive-through line of fast-food places—and most of us have dozens to choose from.

Even people who eat alone might hurry through the meal. A lone diner might eat while reading, elbow propped on a book to keep the page open. Or the television or radio might provide further distraction. These days whole families eat with the television on as background, which works against a relaxed, social atmosphere.

Frankly, other societies think the American way of eating is rather bizarre. Food is everywhere, but we seldom take time to enjoy it, sniffing it before we eat, noticing the individual flavors, chewing each bite well, and relaxing. Eating is supposed to be pleasurable, and most cultures create rituals around food, from the way it looks when it's served to the sequence of each course. For many of us, though, a leisurely dinner is a distant memory. Break-fast with the family is unknown to some people—even on the weekends.

Many weight loss experts believe that this fast-paced eating tends to make us eat more because we eat without thinking and want to eat again soon because we experienced little enjoyment during our meal. There is no doubt some-thing to this idea. But it is also possible that eating slowly and chewing well is good for the satiety mechanism because odor molecules have more time to do their work.

Cindy and Alice, the two single mothers I described in

the previous chapter, discussed many issues around food and eating habits. Both women agreed that meal times had become a struggle to get their kids to settle down and enjoy each other at the dinner table. Both were used to eating breakfast and lunch quickly, and every meal time was filled with distractions. They knew there was something wrong with their patterns, but they also were aware that they couldn't change everything overnight.

In addition to using the odor devices before every meal, they began chewing their food well, and both noticed that others at the table had cleaned their plates before they were half finished. But they kept their resolve to slow down, and eventually, the kids began to eat their meals more slowly, too. At least once a week, the two women planned dinners at each other's house in order to bring their families together and have a more social atmosphere around the table.

Cindy commented that at one time she believed she should work at not enjoying food very much—it was her goal! She thought that if food had little appeal and meals were consumed quickly, then she'd forget about eating. It had never worked that way, of course, but she thought that was only because she had failed to accomplish this "worthy" goal. Nothing could be further from the truth. We are social animals, and food is meant to be tasty, aromatic, and give us great pleasure, often as we share the meals with others. People who lose their appetites through serious illness or reduced ability to smell are at a terrible disadvantage. Sometimes even the social aspect of meals is lost.

Cindy and Alice found that over the long run, they actually ate less because they slowed down and savored each bite. Great resistance to this advice is common because people say they are too busy or don't want to "waste" time eating and on and on. But almost every weight loss expert agrees that chewing food well and slowing the pace of eating is advantageous. Besides, we'd do well to examine exactly what we mean by wasting time. Is spending time with friends or family really such a waste?

These Bubbles Aren't as Ridiculous as They Sound

After chewing a mouthful of food well, try blowing bubbles in it, like blowing bubbles with bubble gum. This sounds very silly, but there is value to this advice. When you blow bubbles in food you are mixing the air and the food molecules, which in turn releases the odor molecules and stimulates the satiety center. I am tempted to recommend that you do this only in the privacy of your own home, but on the other hand, if enough people start blowing bubbles in their food right out in public, then it could become quite fashionable, and who am I to stop a trend?

Learn to Like It Hot

The natural odor in food is more efficiently released when food is hot rather than cold. For example, hot soups and stews are more aromatic than most salads and cold dishes. We have seen in our research that eating hot, aromatic soup before a meal often results in eating less of the main course.

Cindy and Alice also experimented with the hot food idea. You see, once they started losing weight and didn't feel deprived, they were willing to experiment with these other tips. They told us that they began having a "cooking" Sunday about once a month, during which they spent the afternoon making vegetable and bean soups at one of the women's homes. Cindy and Alice shared their concoctions and froze large quantities of nutritious soup and had it available throughout the month. These two women are a good example of the way weight loss led to a new outlook, and even a new lifestyle.

The Fresher the Better

It's best to choose fresh food over packaged or canned. The odor of fresh vegetables is stronger than the odor of canned or frozen vegetables. The same is true for fruit. Dieters are often advised to eat a whole orange or apple instead of drinking the juice made from the fruit. The rationale is that fruit juices have more calories than a piece of fruit. This is true, and in addition, the natural odor in the fruit is available to the olfactory bulb longer than the odor of the juice. This is not because the fruit drink lacks inherent odor, but because it is usually quickly swallowed, and therefore, the aroma does not reach the satiety center.

Pour on Those Herbs and Spices

In general, choose the most aromatic foods possible in order to get the most odor to the olfactory bulb. When we are trying to stimulate appetite among those who suffer from lack of smell, we recommend that they eat hot, spicy foods. People tend to lose weight more quickly and with less feeling of deprivation if they eat food with strong aromas and, therefore, strong taste.

Eating bland foods goes along with our tendency to eat on the run. I recommend avoiding typical vending machine food. It is usually tasteless because it must be refrigerated to keep it fresh. I also suggest eating the more heavily flavored version of "plain" foods. For example, if you eat popcorn, eat the cheese-flavored variety, or choose an onion bagel over a plain one.

Most dieters avoid ethnic restaurants because they believe they won't be able to find their "allowed" foods. But, by encouraging them to eat a wide variety of foods, including spicy dishes, our study participants were free to join their friends at the newest ethnic restaurants and never needed to mention to others that they were trying to lose weight.

They used the smell device before eating, ordered the most aromatic foods, and took home the leftovers.

Most of our participants felt free, sometimes for the first time in their "dieting" lives, to add variety to their meals, rather than eliminate it. Many found that they were noticing aromas and subtle flavors as they never had before. On top of that, they ate less food at each meal but enjoyed it more. Mary Lou, a woman who had been raised on what she said was very "plain" food, lost weight slowly but steadily with the smell devices and began experimenting with dishes she'd never tried before. When she ate in a restaurant, she ordered spicy food, much to the surprise of her husband. Of course, no one could believe she was on a "diet." How could a person who was losing weight possibly eat such a variety of food—and exotic (to her) food at that? They began to believe when they saw her new clothes and noticed how much more energy she had. Again, food is meant to be enjoyed. Sniff away and experiment. You might be surprised how much your eating preferences change as you lose weight.

I Don't Have Room on My Plate

Try limiting your food choices at any one meal. We still encourage variety, but not necessarily all at one time. We have found that people who want to lose weight should eat only two or three different foods during a meal rather than eating a little bit of many foods.

Some of you might be thinking that other cultures, the Japanese for example, do exactly the opposite of what I am recommending, and obesity isn't a serious problem there or throughout Asia. While it is true that the typical Japanese meal includes a wide variety of smells and tastes, the portion of each individual dish is very small. If we could manage this in our culture, it might be advantageous for those who want to—or must—lose weight. However, the typical American meal usually includes larger amounts of each food than we need, and eating fewer kinds of foods may counteract the consequences of our custom.

Who Thought Up "All You Can Eat?"

Avoid buffet tables and "all you can eat" food bars. Even salad bars can be dangerous. Avoid any situation with numerous choices and unlimited quantities. Most people are not able to take one bite of everything, even when they are watching their weight. Even with a smell device, too many selections and unlimited choices spell potential overeating. Lavish buffet tables usually include many food items you like, and following the above advice about limiting variety in each meal is almost impossible.

We also tend to believe, in our culture anyway, that we must get our money's worth. Some of our patients have told us that they feel obligated to load their plates in order not to waste the money they have spent. One of the typical rationales is that they will then eat a light dinner, so the lunch buffet is actually saving them money. It doesn't work that way.

First Bite, Best Bite

We are more sensitive to the smell and taste of our food when we first start eating. When we're distracted by television or reading, we miss the most enjoyable part of the meal. So, in addition to sniffing food before you eat, taking small bites and chewing them well, eat especially slowly at the beginning of a meal. Avoid distractions and concentrate on the way each bite tastes. If you have three different foods on your plate, take a bite of each separately. Many of us have forgotten to savor each individual taste. As you continue eating, your enjoyment of the food diminishes. The first bite of garlic roasted chicken or the rare steak you like is the most enjoyable. We tend to forget this because we usually rush through our meals.

The Dairy Question

While the odor of food stimulates the "I am full" signal in the hypothalamus, one important exception exists—milk. I believe that people who want to lose weight should avoid dairy products because the satiety center does not respond in the same way as it does when other categories foods are ingested. There is a good reason for this important exception, and it based on a built-in physiological mechanism.

In infancy, milk is our primary food, and it promotes rapid growth in the first year of life. In order to survive, we need to take in great quantities of milk, and a mother's milk supply is regulated by the amount the infant consumes. Milk is essentially a bland food, without a strong odor. Therefore, the satiety center is not triggered by milk's odor molecules.

It appears that this is a permanent mechanism; it doesn't change with age. As adults, we can eat large amounts of dairy products without getting the "I am full" message. Think about the popular cheese-and-cracker plates commonly served at cocktail parties and at potluck suppers. Have you ever eaten much more cheese than you planned to? And did you seem to eat a large amount of cheese before you began to feel even slightly full? This is a very typical experience. It's not unusual for one person to eat up to half a pound of cheese without a hint of fullness. The same is true for ice cream; many people are astonished by the amount of ice cream they are able to consume without feeling full.

We are told we need to eat dairy products because we need the calcium. This advice is emphasized for women because their calcium requirements are higher. Obviously, it is important to balance the need for calcium with the advice to avoid dairy foods when trying to lose weight. Many of the commercial diet programs limit dairy products to skim milk, a recommendation that I favor. (Skim milk is not recommended for small children, however.)

Many other foods are rich in calcium, including sardines, salmon, many green leafy vegetables, asparagus, broccoli, oats, and some varieties of nuts and seeds. Most adults can meet their need for calcium without including dairy products in their diets. Those who have milk allergies are accustomed to eating calcium-rich foods and taking calcium supplements if necessary. I recommend that people who want to lose weight generally avoid dairy products, even the reduced-fat or fat-free varieties.

The Problem with Those Diet Sodas

Diet sodas were created to provide the taste of sugared drinks, but without the unwanted calories. The soft drink industry has done an outstanding job of recreating the familiar sweet taste of soft drinks—so outstanding that, in addition to fooling your taste buds, artificial sweeteners can fool your brain as well.

When you drink soda sweetened with sugar and corn sweeteners, the taste causes your brain to interpret the message correctly—you have eaten sugar. It then tells the pancreas to release insulin.(This is technically known as the cephalopancreatic reflex.) The insulin causes your blood sugar level to drop to normal levels. This is the mechanism that is faulty in people who have diabetes.

When you drink artificially sweetened soda, your brain still sends the message to release insulin. But, because you haven't actually ingested sugar, your blood sugar level is not elevated. But the insulin causes your already normal blood sugar level to drop. When blood sugar levels become low, you become hungry, and then you have a tendency to eat more. So you take in extra calories, sometimes far more than you would if you'd had the regular soda rather than the diet variety.

I recommend avoiding drinking artificially sweetened soda with your food. If you must have a diet drink, have it after you've had a full meal. Better yet, switch to flavored, but nonsweetened club soda or mineral water with a slice of lemon or lime. These usually satisfy you just as well as sodas—once you've broken the habit of needing something sweet.

Looking Ahead

I predict that by the year 2010, odorizing our environments to help control appetite will be routine. Research in this area is flourishing, and in a short time, we will understand more completely the mechanism that triggers the desire to eat and the mechanism that tells us when we have had enough. It is possible that we will be able to work with our evolutionary realities and use our natural systems, built in to help us survive, to aid us in maintaining normal body weight.

The combination of physiological, genetic, and psychological research may soon solve the mystery of obesity. For now, we have to work with the tools we have available, and the sense of smell is one the tools we can most easily explore in our daily lives. Take any or all of the advice above. Experiment, and find the tips that work for you.

5 Rebounding— Or Why It's So Tough to Lose Weight

Shirley is fifty-three years old and has been overweight most of her life. "The only time I maintained a normal weight," she told us, "was during the few brief months after I reached my goal weight and ended another diet. Gradually, at first, but then more quickly, the weight started to come back— again. This happened every time I dieted. I'd say I've been a normal weight for a total of eighteen months since age twenty-three or so."

Elizabeth, age thirty-eight, tells a similar story: "I managed to maintain a normal weight as long as I stayed healthy and able to be active. But then I broke my ankle and that set me back. I gained the first twenty-five pounds while my ankle was in a cast. I became active again, but the weight dropped very slowly. So, I went to a commercial diet center, reached my goal weight, and thought I had the problem licked. Then I had major surgery, and two years after that, I had a bout with pneumonia that kept me immobile for over two months. My weight climbed and climbed and as much as I resisted another diet, I had no choice. I tried a liquid fasting program but as soon as my weight was normal again, the numbers on the scales started to get bigger and bigger. Diets are a nightmare—and even worse, they have kept me in yo-yo mode for twenty years."

These stories are so familiar that almost every person who has ever dieted can identify with them. Almost no one is able to go on a diet, lose weight, and keep it off for a long period of time. In controlled studies, it was found that almost all the weight a dieter lost on commercial or self-directed diets is regained within five years. That's why we don't call our system of using odors a diet. We are convinced that diets don't work, will never work, and that to put people on them is cruel and sets them up for failure.

The rebound effect is real and powerful. It's what the yo-yo syndrome is all about. Weight loss, followed by weight gain, followed by more weight loss, and usually even more weight gain. That's why we often see people becoming increasingly overweight as they get older. Those "few pounds more" each time weight is gained add up over the years.

I understand why people are taken in again and again by the promises each new diet makes. Some women have told me that they buy every magazine with a headline that says, "Get Ready for Summer [or winter] Lose 10 Pounds in Two Weeks." Each time, they approach the article with hope. Overweight people in our culture are vulnerable to scraps of hope. But very little new material is available in the diet industry—except for medication, which has problems of its own. For the most part, the information offered is a rehash of old diets. Once we understand the rebound effect, we won't believe wild claims, and we won't fall for diets that promise that we'll lose interest in food. (That's an unhealthy hope anyway.)

When people start a liquid fasting diet, for example, most are generally pleased that weight loss is rapid at first, and almost miraculously, they don't miss eating. But they haven't learned new ways to eat, and in addition, they're metabolic rate has slowed down because the body is hoarding calories. The body is reacting to faminelike conditions, and when it starts receiving food, it doesn't rev up, so to speak, just because the "famine" is over. Most people find that the old cravings are back in short order.

Sound physiological reasons exist for the difficulties people encounter when they diet. The rebound effect has nothing to do with will power, and as we'll see, it's the natural consequence of attempting to ignore basic drives and physiology.

Mental Resolve versus Physiological Realities

Earlier, I talked about the ventral medial nucleus of the hypothalamus, the satiety center, which provides the signal that we are full—satisfied—and should stop eating. The hypothalamus is the master gland in that it regulates many functions, such as body temperature, metabolic rate, blood pressure, and so forth. These functions are unconscious—operating, for the most part, outside our conscious control. We don't think about regulating our temperature, and we don't consciously have to keep our hearts pumping blood through our bodies.

The regulatory functions of the hypothalamus give us a clue about why diets almost always fail. When we look at the body and learn how it functions, it becomes obvious that diets usually are counterproductive and lead to weight gain in the long run. Most people are resistant to this idea. They think that if they only muster up enough will power, the next diet will work. We call this the "one more diet syndrome," because it usually goes along with statements like these:

- "I can feel it—I'm ready. This time my diet will work."

- "This diet promises that I'll feel full because of certain foods I have to eat every day. That's been the missing link. I can go for one more diet—especially this one."

- "This diet is all about the right combination of foods—it's totally different from my other diets. That's why this time it will work—I *will* lose weight."

- "I've never weighed my food before—that's what makes this diet different. I'm sure it will work if I put my mind to it. Weighing my food will give me something to do instead of just focusing on the food."

- "This diet isn't really a diet, because you don't eat food, which will be better for me. If I can eliminate the need to eat, I'll be okay. Just drinking liquid is actually easier. Eventually, they say, I'll lose my appetite, and food will be repulsive to me. When I do start eating regular meals again, it won't have any appeal— sounds good to me."

Most people in our weight loss studies all had "one more diet" stories. Each new diet has something that's just a little different, and that difference leads to wishful thinking. It's erroneous to assume that a diet can change our basic drives, drives that have served us well for millions of years.

Dieting Is a Lot Like Trying to Go without Sleep

To talk about the rebound effect in relation to eating can be an emotionally charged topic. To take it out of the emotional realm, let's look at an analogous drive, our need for sleep. You can't help being tired, even if you will yourself to stay awake. If you stay up all night, you're bound to be tired during the day, and the next night you'll probably go to bed early. If you stay up for two full days, you can barely stay awake. Sure, you have little spurts of energy now and again. You may drink strong coffee and get a caffeine rush, or you exercise, splash cold water in your face, turn on the television for distraction, and a try a host of other things to stay awake. But the fact is that the human body is programmed to sleep at night. Eventually, you can't overcome this need, no matter what you do.

If you overwork and cheat yourself of rest, you will probably sleep more the first chance you get. Your body demands rest—at some point—you can't fight it, and one way or another, you will get the rest you need. That's why people often sleep later on weekends, especially if they stay up late during the week. During the 1996 Summer Olympic Games, reporters did "people on the street" interviews and polls and asked people if they were tired during the day because they stayed up to watch the popular track and field or gymnastic events at night. Large numbers of people admitted that they were becoming sleep deprived, when night after night they resisted going to bed because they didn't want to miss their favorite events. Almost all said that they would make up their lost sleep on the weekend. I wonder if productivity figures were down during the two weeks of extensive—and very late—Olympic Games coverage. When we try to go against our natural physiological tendencies, there are consequences, and we may not like them.

Most of us try to fit thirty hours of activity into a twenty-four-hour day, and many people talk about being tired virtually all the time. This is another phenomenon that puzzles people from other cultures. We gulp our food, work around the clock, and cram our calendars with one event after another. Then we wonder why we're overweight, tired, and stressed out. Most of us are so used to this pace that we have forgotten that there is another way to live. And I plead guilty, too. I'm not trying to point a finger at anyone else here. I just suggest that we would do well to reevaluate the way we live in this very hectic society.

When we give into sleep after a period of deprivation, we tend to sleep not only longer, but deeper—reaching stage 3 or 4 sleep. When we talk about sleeping soundly and deeply, we've reached these stages. Ask any mother who must stay up with a baby all night what kind of sleep she experiences when she finally gets a chance to rest. She may even wake up groggy, which often indicates deep sleeping. The same situation occurs when we stay up late studying for finals or working on a project. When we finally sleep, we experience a *rebound* effect because we sleep more than we normally would. Those of you who have been on many diets recognize the rebound effect all too well, but you may blame yourself for it. To me, this is analogous to blaming yourself because you need more sleep at night.

The human need to sleep during the night probably is a result of evolutionary development. Given the fact that our night vision isn't as good as that of other animals, we would be in more danger if we did our hunting and gathering in the dark. In the Darwinian theory of survival of the fittest, we probably have a built-in mechanism that makes sleeping at night and carrying out our other activities during the day natural to us.

We even need regular exposure to light for a part of the brain to function normally. Evidence suggests that night-shift workers are more susceptible to infection, sleep disorders, and even depression because their natural biological rhythm—the circadian rhythm—is interrupted. Seasonal Affective Disorder (SAD) is linked with the relative lack of exposure to sunlight during the darker winter months. Certainly, individuals vary, and some people adjust to night work very well. Still, generally speaking, our bodies are programmed for daylight activity and rest during the darkest hours.

Our ability to gain weight and store body fat also has, as I've said, evolutionary significance. Our species would have become extinct long ago had we not been able to adjust to periods when food was scarce and to eat more when food was plentiful.

It's almost unheard of for an animal living in its natural environment to become obese. Yet, once we domesticate animals, they are at risk of eating too much, too, and we may even put our dogs and cats on a "lean cuisine" regimen. Many of our pets have unlimited access to food and are less physically active than they would be if they lived in the wild—just like us. So, it's no wonder that our pets gain weight right along with us.

When people are on deprivation diets, the body reacts as if food is scarce. Then, when food is plentiful again, the brain sends a signal to eat, eat, eat—probably more than we want or need to—we rebound, and make up for the period of deprivation. So, if we deprive ourselves of sleep, the body eventually rebounds and demands that we rest, often in long, deep periods of sleep. If we deprive ourselves of food, the body eventually demands that we eat. The body doesn't know when that next period of scarcity will be, so to protect us from starvation, it urges us to fill up, store fat, and survive. So much for the wisdom of "starvation" diets. These diets don't work *with* nature; they work against it.

One of the study subjects told us that her grandmother was considered a real beauty in her small, mid-western town. "It seems odd, too," she said, "because by today's standards she was fat. They really did call it pleasingly plump back then. During the Great Depression, my grandmother's weight was practically a status symbol."

I'm sure that this woman is correct—her grandmother's family was relatively well off during the Depression, a time whent food was scarce for many Americans. We must remember that we live in just about the only society ever to consider extreme thinness a sign of beauty. Extreme thinness is like fighting to stay awake for days at a time. It's just not the way nature designed us to be.

From Admiration to Contempt

A lot of room exists for normalcy between extreme thinness and the obesity we see rampant today. Being severely overweight poses a significant health risk, and obesity is brought on by affluence and year-round availability of food. But obesity is also an inevitable result of the rebound effect—too much deprivation followed by overeating. Our bodies haven't adjusted to our new situation; however, our own primal instincts urge us to overeat despite the health risks. It's as if we're in the midst of an evolutionary transition, which on the one hand could favor thin people. But it's also possible we are experiencing a temporary abundance of food that could be reversed at any time, in which case the ability to store fat will continue to be favored in evolutionary development.

Although I would never encourage anyone to attempt to live up to the superthin image of today's models and movie stars (many of the latter need body doubles in movies because even they don't meet the standard of perfection demanded), I do encourage obese people to lose excess pounds and keep them off. It is possible to avoid the re-bound effect by working with the body rather than fighting its drives. If we eliminate deprivation diets, we eliminate the rebound effect. Rebounding is the underlying cause of the yo-yo syndrome, and we can't continue to put people on diets that start them on this insidious cycle.

That said, the physical consequences of obesity, not to mention the emotional ones, are too great to ignore. For reasons from the increased risk of hypertension (high blood pressure), stroke, and heart disease to the stress on joints in the ankles and knees, obesity must be addressed.

It's extremely important to me, however, that we address the problem as a physiological one and not as a matter of character weakness. You see, in addition to being a ma-terialistic society, where all material items, including food, are viewed as good, we are also a culture that respects rational, cognitive abilities and tries to downplay basic drives and emotions.

Our drives are not part of our intellectual capacities, however, so we often view them as a liability rather than the reason we are able to survive. A basic misunderstanding about human drives is partially responsible for the contempt we have in our society for overweight people.

Even normal-weight persons sometimes express guilt when they are hungry. Some people, especially those who believe they can and must control everything, don't like admitting that they are tired—they believe it's the same as saying they are weak. We have little respect for human physiological needs, although we acknowledge them in other animals, including our close primate cousins. We have foolishly decided that since we have the ability to think and reason, we are no longer members of the animal kingdom. Thinking of our natural drives as liabilities rather than assets has led to the ludicrous situation of judging obesity as a sign that the person lacks moral courage or strength of character.

Much of what we do in our society actually works against our internal drives. We believe that sheer will power should be able to overcome these troublesome needs—even the need to eat or sleep. We set one standard, apply it to everyone, and those who can't meet it are considered failures. How many adolescents are called lazy because they need more sleep than others? How many overweight people are called lazy because they can't lose weight?

One of my patients said that we're "schizophrenic" about our drives, however. We try to regulate eating, sleeping, and even sex. But media images are filled with sexual images, the restaurant industry is booming, and sweets are promoted as one of life's basic pleasures. For example, in the midst of this sensory barrage, we send a message that the sexual drive should be acted on only under carefully regulated circumstances. We live in a society obsessed with sex, but we then regulate sexual activity, even to the point that we pass laws that make some sexual acts between consenting adults a crime. We worship foods like chocolate, but we tell some people that they're morally weak if they eat chocolate cake. And then we wonder why, given our basic physiology and our cultural norms, people have a difficult time losing weight.

All these mixed messages led me to believe that deprivation diets, food plans, lists of foods our patients should eat or should always avoid, were futile. After the results of our study, I believe this even more strongly. The beauty of using the odors is that normal life can go on. More than anything else, this seemed to make an important difference to people choosing to try this weight loss and weight control method.

Rebounding Is Painful

One of the worst consequences of the rebound effect is the emotional toll it takes on dieters. Here they are, working so hard for so long to eat so little. Their bodies are desperately trying to stay the same, so each pound lost seems like a battle that has been fought and won. Deprivation diets tend to lead to fatigue, which sets the person up to be discouraged and without energy to sustain a normal life. Every ounce of will power is usually necessary to stay on a severely restrictive diet, and sometimes the person will become socially isolated. This is an emotionally painful process, made worse by the rebound that inevitably occurs.

Bob, one of study participants described it this way: "The rebound started when I went on vacation with my brother. We went with a tour group to several Mediterranean countries, where we were served sumptuous lunches and dinners every night. The first few days I tried to turn away from the food, but I eventually thought if I just ate moderately, I could get back on my diet when I returned home. But once I started eating normally—like others on the tour—I was out of control. I kept eating more and more. Each day I resolved to stop, but each day I would fail. I felt hungry, that's what was so strange. It was as if my body was demanding food—more and more food. It was a great trip, but I was emotionally down for weeks after I returned home.

I didn't want to go back to the office because I was sure the people I worked with were talking about me—'Here comes Bob, he failed *again*,' or 'We knew he couldn't do it—he doesn't have the will power to lose weight.' I guess they're right, but I have to do something or I'll be unhappy for the rest of my life."

If Bob had tried to stay awake for five days, no one would have faulted him for falling asleep. If he'd talked about jet lag, a natural physiological response to disruptions to our internal time clock, no one would have said he was weak. However, few people, except those who have experienced it, understand how deep Bob's feelings of self-loathing and weakness went.

Bob has done very well on our program. He has succeeded in "tricking" his body, so to speak, and has not experienced a rebound effect. He has made the smell devices part of his life, and he doesn't count calories or fat grams, weigh his food, or skip every piece of cake that comes his way. Bob lost weight over a period of months and added exercise to his life, and now his body has adjusted to a new weight. As long as Bob understands what rebounding is, he will never deprive himself of basic sustenance again.

Set Point, Homeostasis, and Exercise

The hypothalamus is designed to help the body stay the same. It's as if it gets used to certain conditions and fights to keep them just the way they are. Part of rebounding and the difficulty in keeping weight off is linked with homeostasis, which essentially means maintaining the status quo. When we talk about set point, we're really talking about a weight that the body is used to and struggles, often against our better judgment, to maintain.

Years of dieting have shown that weight can be lost; those same years of dieting have revealed the rebound effect and have given scientists another issue over which to puzzle.

The concept of a set point, a weight the body has decided is normal, is now widely accepted. The problem is, how do we change the set point when the natural tendency is toward homeostasis?

Slow weight loss is certainly one way to help the body adapt to a lower weight because it gives the body a chance to readjust the set point. Diets designed to take weight off rapidly work against this adaptation, which is one reason our foundation decided against any kind of food plan in our study. We also didn't have goals for how rapidly weight should be lost. In other words, we looked for slow, steady weight loss, rather than celebrating over big numbers. True, some of our study subjects did lose pounds rapidly, but we didn't design the program that way.

I mention this because I don't want you to be discouraged if you lose only a pound a week, or 4 or 5 pounds a month. You are helping your body adjust to a lower weight, which in turn helps to fight the rebounding effect.

So, what about exercise? No doubt exercise plays a role in resetting the set point. In other words, regular exercise changes the weight the body believes is normal. In chapter 8, I discuss exercise and make recommendations. But if you are just starting this program and the thought of heading to the gym or slipping an exercise video into the VCR makes you want to close the book, then don't worry about it right now. Exercise is important, and I believe it is critical to maintaining permanent weight loss, but you don't have to start today.

Some people are surprised by my attitude about this. We didn't include exercise in our study protocol—not because I don't believe in it, but because it would have added a variable, and we wouldn't have had such clear evidence that the odors work so well. But I'm glad we didn't "mandate" it for another, far more important reason. Exercise would have been just another chore, just another diet program concept, and just another way for people to feel like failures.

Many diet programs fail because people can't stick with them. They can't eat special food, feel deprived, and then go for ninety-minute walks, too.

So, if you haven't exercised very much, don't feel pressured to begin immediately. Just start using the odors. Use them frequently, watch yourself leave food on your plate, see some results on the scale, and then you'll probably feel more like moving around. I've seen it happen. The most exercise-resistent people find themselves avid walkers or runners or swimmers once they feel well enough to enjoy physical activity.

6 *Understanding and Beating Cravings*

Marianne was very upset about her inability to fight off cravings, which she described as "constantly with her," a "scourge on her life," and "the bane of her existence. She had cravings for sweets most of the time, but they became especially intense during the two weeks between the ovulatory part of her menstrual cycle and the onset of her period. "There are only a few days a month when the cravings are manageable," she said.

Like many people, Marianne viewed cravings as a sign of weakness. The cravings for chocolate, ice cream, and candy were often so strong that she thought she wouldn't survive without these foods. Because she looked at merely having the cravings as a character flaw, she had engaged in much secret eating during her thirty-five years. In public, she ate about the same amount of food as everyone else, so she did her "shameful" eating alone at home. Over the years, she had become increasingly socially isolated, often leaving gatherings early because she felt compelled to go home and satisfy her cravings. Her weight gain, followed by periodic diets, had left her feeling hopeless. Marianne is a professionally accomplished young woman, but her extra 50 pounds combined with cravings that seemed virtually uncontrollable resulted in very low self-esteem. This is logical, however, as long as we continue to view cravings as a character issue.

Some people crave doughnuts—they say they need two

or three just to start the day—and that their evening isn't complete without cake and ice cream. Other people crave potato chips and dip or french fries, and still others say that the day isn't complete if they don't have a bowl of buttered popcorn. In every case, they describe the need for these foods as a craving. For the most part, people think of cravings as something bad and to be overcome, one way or another. There's only one time in a woman's life when cravings aren't considered a sign of weakness.

When Cravings Are Acceptable

The one time that cravings are socially acceptable is during pregnancy. Movies and television comedies are filled with scenes where a woman asks her husband to get her chocolate ice cream or dill pickles at 2:00 A.M.—taking a quick trip to the convenience store if necessary. In the movies, anyway, men generally give in to this request because when a woman is pregnant, she's considered "special."

One woman we know said she couldn't seem to get enough of a particular kind of chewing gum when she was pregnant and took to buying it in big cartons. Another woman said that she ate coconut cake every day—without guilt. Other women crave various kinds of food, from burgers to butter cookies, and they never know when a craving will "strike."

It's interesting to note, however, that in studies that explored cravings, the number of cravings reported is actually no different during pregnancy than it was before. The difference is that women tend to give in to their cravings during pregnancy because it is socially acceptable to gain weight at that time.

As an aside addressed to readers who expect to become pregnant in the future, I want to emphasize that gaining some weight during pregnancy is healthful—that's the way it's supposed to be. However, our society's emphasis on body image has even extended to pregnancy. When actress Demi Moore appeared pregnant and nude on the cover of *People* magazine, she offered still another new standard for women to live up to.

A generation ago, women routinely gained 30 to 40 pounds during their pregnancies. Later, 20 to 25 pounds was considered a healthful weight gain. But, in recent years, a 5 to 10 pound weight gain is not uncommon. I'm concerned about this emphasis on a "thin" pregnancy because it could have adverse consequences for the developing fetus as well as the mother.

Mother Nature has designed the fetus to be a very efficient "parasite," and if not given sufficient nutrients, the fetus will "steal" them from the mother. This frequently happens when the mother's diet isn't adequate, often because she is attempting to control her weight and is cutting her caloric intake. Many nutrients could be ingested in amounts too small to feed the mother and the fetus. For example, if there isn't enough calcium to meet the needs of the growing fetus, the mineral will be drawn from the mother's bones and teeth. This predisposes the mother to dental problems and earlier onset of osteoporosis (thinning of the bones).

I'm addressing this section to readers whose weight roughly falls within a wide normal range. Morbid obesity during pregnancy is harmful, too, which is why many overweight women are advised to attain a weight within the range of normal before becoming pregnant. Too much weight gain during pregnancy is associated with many health problems, including gestational diabetes. That said, I'm particularly concerned about the phenomenon of a "too thin" pregnancy. When women are pleased when they gain only 3 or 4 pounds during a pregnancy, something is seriously wrong.

Another Way to Tolerate Frustration

As discussed in detail in the next chapter, cravings and overeating often are part of the mechanism we use to tolerate frustration. Some people think of food—or the act of eating—as a way to handle stress and frustration, and satisfying a craving may bring immediate relief. This relief doesn't last long, however, because the issue that led to the episode of overeating doesn't go away. That's why cravings followed by eating followed by cravings are like a cycle that goes on and on and causes a person to feel worse and worse because they feel so bad about overeating. But there may be other ways to explain cravings, leading us back—once again—to the brain.

"I Need that Chemical—NOW"

Scientists have conducted research that suggests that we may crave sweets to increase one of a group of neurotransmitters, chemicals in the brain that regulate many functions, including our mood states. Our bodies produce numerous neurotransmitters, but the one believed to be linked with cravings for sweets is serotonin.

There are drugs (phenfluramine, or Fen-Fen, as it's commonly known, is one) that increase serotonin and, hence, may reduce appetite and cravings. Certain drugs are serotonin agonists, meaning that they help the body produce more of this chemical. Interestingly, Prozac, a drug prescribed for depression, is a serotonin agonist, and one of the side effects reported when this drug was first used was reduction in appetite, often followed by weight loss. This occurred even when patients didn't expect or desire this side effect.

How Does Depression Fit In?

Many overweight people describe themselves as depressed, even to the point of being suicidal. However, often they are not taken seriously because their depression isn't "classic," meaning that it doesn't fit the textbook definition of the illness—and depression is truly an illness. In classic depression, loss of appetite and weight loss are expected symptoms, along with deep disinterest in life, constant crying, inability to carry out normal activities, and so forth.

Many overweight people suffer from "atypical depression," meaning that increased appetite is often present along with other symptoms, most of which are not nearly as severe as those present with classic depression. Indeed, most overweight people function in the world quite normally, have families and jobs, and are involved in the world. They may carry around a deep sadness about their weight, but they generally live at least fairly normal lives. This suggests that eating is a form of "self-treatment," a way to lift mood as well as handle frustration.

However, it's possible that people crave foods, such as chocolate, that contain chemicals that are "precursors" to key neurotransmitters, meaning that the chemicals combine with others chemicals to produce these substances. One important chemical is found in chocolate. It's no wonder that eating chocolate seems like self-medicating—it could be that it is!

Rather than having a character flaw, our study participant Marianne, mentioned at the start of this chapter, may be self-medicating in the most basic way. She is eating foods that will help her produce a neurotransmitter in the brain that she needs to "treat" this atypical depression.

Her cravings increase at mid-cycle, which is a time when some women develop a form of mild depression, called dysthymia. We refer to this as "reduced mood," and it is often characterized by increased cravings for chocolate, suggesting that the body is attempting to get the precursor it needs to produce serotonin. The mild mood alteration may also be experienced as part of the frustration phenomenon, which also leads to cravings for comfort foods. Sweet foods, particularly those containing chocolate, are often high on the list of comfort foods.

How Do Odors Help?

We know that serotonin is one of the neurotransmitters in the olfactory bulb. We also know that using the smell devices can act to interrupt a craving, stop it before it is acted on with the actual food. Chocolate provides an interesting example. If you can't smell chocolate, you can't taste it. If you bite into a chocolate bar while holding your nose, the candy tends to taste like chalk or cardboard. But some of our study subjects told us that just smelling chocolate reduced their craving.

Although we don't know exactly how the odors work to reduce cravings, it's possible that:

- the smell of chocolate, for example, works on the brain and increases serotonin.

- or the odor provides a reasonable substitute or alternative and permits the person to sniff away without eating. In other words, the comfort value of the smell satisfies the cravings.

- or the act of sniffing the odor reduces the craving because it reduces frustration. Using the smell device is a direct substitute for eating.

I Can Pass on the Chocolate, But Bring on the Pizza

Although some people crave a wide variety of foods, most people's cravings fall into one of two broad categories. Some people can pass up sweet food in a minute. They simply don't care about the taste of doughnuts or pastries or ice cream. This group craves fatty, usually salty foods, such as pizza or potato chips. At this point, we don't have a biological reason for this category of craving. The best we can do is speculate that perhaps this "fatty/salty" craving group associates these foods with comfort. Perhaps in their childhood households, these were the foods that were offered when they were frustrated.

While we haven't studied individual responses to odors, we have noticed that, as we've said before, weight loss increases in direct proportion to the amount the smell devices are used. The more people sniffed, the more they lost. People who crave fatty, salty foods probably prefer the devices that contain the smell of pizza or roasting meat. Likewise, those who crave sweet foods most likely reach for the device that contains the Oreo cookie scent or the odor of Good & Plenty candy. It's also possible that those who went through periods of frequent sniffing were craving a particular food, and the scent satisfied that craving without the need to taste the food.

Ways to Break the Craving Habit

Some people beat cravings by eating a small amount of the food that is tempting them. They can take a bite or two of chocolate or a handful of chips, and the craving is gone. Some people can eat fruit as a substitute for the refined sugar found in prepared sweets. I've heard people say that a small amount of fruit juice will cut their cravings immediately.

If this works, I'm all for trying it. But overweight people who can take "just a few bites" are the minority. Most people who can eat that moderately are thin to begin with. Most of the people who are already overweight and experiencing cravings are unable to eat half a candy bar or take two cookies out of the package and save the rest for later.

Many study participants reported that, before they entered our program, they required more sweets or fatty foods as time went on. A patient named Sidney told us that he needed a bigger and bigger "fix" of sugar. He described it as similar to the way he developed the smoking habit as a teenager. As the months went on, he needed an increasing number of cigarettes to satisfy his cravings. He eventually quit smoking, but then he substituted food for smoking. The same pattern repeated itself.

By using the odor device, Sidney went through a process

of retraining himself. He deliberately took a few bites of a dessert, used the inhaler, and pushed the plate away. He didn't keep the foods he craved in his house for several months after he started losing weight with odors. He preferred instead to break his habit of having the food around— literally, under his nose. He had the inhaler to satisfy his nose when he began craving the sugary foods. Over time, he was able to eat the sweets he liked without overeating. He felt more like what he thought of as a "normal" person.

Restriction Sets Up Cravings

In our "sniffing" program, no food restrictions are imposed. Restrictive eating always leads to cravings. People who try to "save" their calories during the day in order to eat a big meal at night are often hit with powerful cravings by mid-afternoon, if not sooner. In these cases, diet soda often intensifies the cravings, and the person ends up eating whatever is handy, usually gulping it down, hardly noticing the taste. This is another reason that diets often lead to rebounding, and the rebounding pattern is usually initiated with cravings. Because the person has been so restricted, they can't seem to get enough ice cream or potato chips or whatever the craving centered on.

The exact mechanisms that produce all cravings aren't yet known, but I believe we will find that brain chemistry plays a big role. The best way to avoid intense cravings is by eating a wide variety of foods, eating regular meals, and getting plenty of rest. Cravings are always worse when one is tired or frustrated.

New Habits, New Insights

Sometimes people worry about becoming addicted to sniffing the odors, the way they feel addicted to the foods they crave. What they are actually doing, however, is breaking the habit of craving food and developing the habit of sniffing. Whether this switch in habits is possible because of the way the odors act on the brain or simply from a behavioral response, it is essentially replacing a harmful habit with one that is harmless in and of itself and is a good substitute for caloric and fat-laden foods.

In the process of losing weight with odor devices, many people are able to stop their cravings and their tendency to overeat for long periods of time. This enables them to gain insight and clarity about the unconscious drives that are part of the reason they eat in the first place. If people form the habit of sniffing while they learn about themselves and attain a healthier weight, then I don't see the harm.

Many of our study participants have gained a deeper understanding of the concept of frustration and the way human beings learn to cope. One thing is sure, overweight people aren't inherently weak, and they don't have character flaws. Many simply have developed a habitual cycle of over-eating that is experienced as cravings.

I recommend that you use the odors as much as you want to when you start this program. Monitor your cravings—some of our patients keep a journal, as I've mentioned. If the odor of cookies cuts your craving and prevents you from grabbing a half dozen cookies out of the package, then note that in your journal. Write down how you feel when you've successfully avoided the foods that you once craved almost daily.

As you continue to use smells and you're eating less, you'll note the times that you have the urge to use odors. If you're like most people, you'll begin to see a pattern, one that has probably taken a lifetime to develop. In the next chapter, we'll explore the concept of frustration and how we learn, from the time we are infants, to handle it.

7 Our Emotions Can't Be Ignored

Some of our study participants have a difficult time admitting that they eat in search of emotional well-being, or at least to influence how they feel from moment to moment or hour to hour. When they were first interviewed, many were ashamed to tell us that food gave them comfort or settled their nerves or even helped them get their mind off problems in their lives. Eating for emotional reasons is neither unusual nor shameful, however, because most people reach for food, at least some of the time, motivated by a desire to satisfy an emotional need. Some people just pay a bigger price in weight gain than others. Physiological differences play a role in the unfortunate fact that some people gain weight by overeating while their thin counterparts don't.

Lori, age twenty-eight, maintained a normal weight throughout college and law school. She was then hired by a prestigious law firm in San Francisco, and the pressure was on. "I gained twenty pounds during the first six months and another thirty after that. I couldn't seem to control my eating—I began munching on snack food even when I wasn't hungry. That was new for me." The realization that she was eating for comfort was gradual.

Eventually, she began to see the connection between her emotional needs and reaching for food. She said that food thoughts and fantasies began to dominate even when the snack food supplies ran out. She became anxious, the same way smokers may become anxious when they are down to the last cigarette in their pack. Finally, she realized how much anxiety she was experiencing over her performance on her first legal job. In addition, she worked such long hours that she had little opportunity to do anything except "sleep a little, eat a lot, and work."

Marilyn, age fifty, also described eating when she was nervous or tense. She taught English in a very large, over-crowded, and professionally demanding high school. As if that weren't enough, she was going through a very painful divorce. "I eat a big lunch, snack on my breaks, and stop for a muffin on the way home. Then I eat ice cream and snack until it's time for bed. I've even gone out at night to get the foods that I'm craving so much. But it doesn't make sense. I'm not hungry, but I eat anyway and now I'm gaining weight."

Our study participants have joked that sometimes they eat because they are nervous or unhappy, and then when conditions improve in their lives, they eat to celebrate because they are happy and excited. In other words, no single emotion triggers the urge to eat. And eating in response to emotional states is part of the mechanism that causes obesity. But it's important to reiterate that emotions and food are linked for the vast majority of the population.

It's a Frustrating World

From the time we were infants, we were set on a developmental course through which we learned to regulate our bodily functions and our response to emotional frustrations. Just as we adjust to society's expectations and learn to regulate bladder and bowel functions, we also learn to control frustration. The better we are at moderating our responses to frustration, the more successful we are in school, our careers, and in relationships.

I am using frustration as a general term for emotional states, both conscious and unconscious, that affect every human being. I'm defining frustration broadly here. It might include irritation, boredom, impatience, tension, or anxiety. We may be frustrated when we think others don't understand us or aren't giving us the attention we need. We may be frustrated when we overwork, and a project seems to have no end. We may be frustrated that our clothes don't fit and, paradoxically, seek food as a way to relieve our self-disgust. Day in and day out, we experience frustration.

In infancy, we are frustrated, and the people taking care of us may not know why. We make our first link between food and comfort when we have a nipple or a bottle thrust in our mouths because we are crying. When we don't know what's wrong with a baby, it's our natural tendency to assume that he or she must be hungry. We're often wrong, but we keep trying it anyway.

Later, when we're toddlers, we may be comforted with food when we're fussy or to divert us from some forbidden activity. Parents lure a toddler away from the china cabinet by using food as the bait. Statements like, "Come and have a cookie" or "Here comes Grandpa with ice cream," imprint the idea in our minds that food is a way to moderate our frustration. Many a temper tantrum has been stopped in its tracks with candy or cookies. And, as will become clear, this cycle often begins in response to fatigue.

As we become adults, the cycle continues and the connection between relieving frustration and eating is set for life. We may not admit that we'd like to have a temper tantrum, but we reach for the comfort food all the same. And the thing is, it works—at least temporarily. For a period of time, we forget the frustration and concentrate on other things. Just like toddlers, we don't have the temper tantrum because we're munching on chips, candy, ice cream, or popcorn.

It's not surprising that we may overeat when we're

excited or happy, too. After all, most societies have rituals for celebrations and happy occasions. Almost all celebrations and social gatherings are planned around food, from a Thanksgiving feast to the July Fourth barbecue, not to mention weddings and birthday parties.

When people eat to relieve frustration, they often use the same substance they connect with comfort in childhood. Some people say that their comfort foods—those foods they crave when they are tense, anxious, sad, or angry—are the same ones they ate as children. Internally, we associate solving the problem with eating the food. Eat ice cream, calm down. Eat cookies, and the tension is gone.

Most of us know that over the long run, we don't solve a problem by eating—it's an illusion. Just as alcohol doesn't solve a feeling of inadequacy or make family or financial problems go away, food doesn't solve anything either. Smoking, nail-biting, and all the other habits we develop are, in essence, ways we have adopted to temper frustration.

If we were rational beings only, devoid of emotional capacity, we could say, "This isn't working—I better find a different way." Ultimately, people do quit drinking or stop smoking and break the nail-biting habit, but often it takes more than one attempt, and they may be very uncomfortable during the process of "withdrawing" from the habit. Then, too, they try to substitute another way to modulate frustration, and for many people food becomes the most available—and socially acceptable—choice. A former smoker may start overeating, and recovering alcoholics often gain weight, especially if they have quit smoking, too. This is discouraging, of course, since people work hard to break addictions, often because they want to experience improved health. To then gain weight can be extremely frustrating. Some of our study participants told us about their struggles to achieve better health—and avoid serious problems—only to find themselves with 30 or 40 pounds they don't need.

Sometimes it isn't the food that relieves the frustration,

but the act of eating itself. Think about the cluster of people around buffet tables at business or social functions. Much of the eating is a response to nervousness, perhaps because we don't know very many people at the event. We're expected to be relaxed and sociable, but we may feel anxious and tense. The physical act of munching on cheese and crackers helps us relax and feel as if we fit in.

Throughout human history, we've tended to eat in groups. Eating dinner alone in our own apartments or ordering lunch to eat by ourselves at our desks actually goes against our "herd" instinct. When we eat in groups, particularly with people we know, we often eat more because we are sociable and usually happier (although the odor devices counteract that tendency while allowing us to participate in the social aspect of the gathering).

In social settings filled with strangers, we may even experience fear, which induces what we call the sympathetic, or fight or flight, response—the source of what makes us anxious and hyperalert. An animal in the wild is in this fight or flight response when he rushes to kill that day's food source. When he is eating his captured prey, however, he is in the parasympathetic response, which is a relaxed state. Eating when we're anxious is our human way of converting from the stressful, hyperalert state to a more relaxed mood. People rushing around their offices, working hard to get a project finished to meet a deadline, are in this hyperalert state. No wonder they overeat when the day finally ends. Unconsciously, they know it's a reliable way to relax, not so different from the animals in the forest. Consciously, however, they may just feel weak. If they attempt to justify their eating, they'll call it a "reward" and usually feel weak anyway.

Many people's behavior while flying provides another good illustration of the connection between food and anxiety. Many people are anxious before takeoff, but they relax more when the snack or meal is served. Very few people turn down the offer of a beverage or food on a plane, even if they are neither thirsty nor hungry. We interviewed flight attendants who told us that when passengers were provided with a carry-on bag lunch, many—if not most—people started eating before the plane left the runway. Again, the unconscious is at work, attempting to induce relaxation in a situation where anxieties abound.

Food is not the only way we change behavior in response to fear. Some people tap their feet or say a prayer or hum a particular song before boarding a plane (or giving a speech or entering a room full of strangers). Other people immediately start working or reading the minute they settle into their seat. All these activities are ways to divert attention from the fear or anxiety they're experiencing. They may not be conscious that they're repeating a fear-reducing habit, one they developed for just such occasions. We could say that eating is a nearly universal method of relieving frustration, and all the other habits reflect individual tendencies.

Some people relieve the frustration that comes with loneliness by compensating with food. Much overeating is done when alone. Many of our study participants have described food as their "friend." Smokers say the same thing about cigarettes. Sometimes a traumatic event such as a divorce, or the death of a significant person, or even a job change starts the cycle of isolation through food. As these people become more isolated, they then eat more because they are even lonelier. This becomes a vicious cycle and is very difficult to break. The odor devices, however, can break the cycle by providing a substitute for the food, which leads to weight loss, often leading to reaching out to others and becoming more active and involved in the world. We know that, tough as it is, most people are capable of breaking destructive habits and cycles. There is always reason to hope, and insight can lead to action.

Odors May Help Us Cope

Psychotherapy and support groups often help relieve serious emotional overeating difficulties. Gaining insight into why we reach for food can be helpful and alleviate the suffering caused by these overeating and weight gain cycles. I encourage people to seek professional help or a self-help group if they are in great pain over an emotionally based overeating problem. Too often, the overweight suffer in silence, some even believing that their problem is simply one of will power, and therefore, they don't deserve help. Nonsense. We all deserve help when we experience difficulties that we haven't been able to handle alone. In many other societies, the individualism to which we have become accustomed, and indeed promote, in many ways would be unthinkable.

Because eating in response to frustration is a nearly universal phenomenon, begun in infancy and carried over to adulthood, it makes sense to explore ways to minimize frustration or modulate it in a constructive way. We can develop strategies that help us refrain from reaching for the nearest candy bar or going off in search of food for reasons we don't completely understand.

Much of our research about odors and emotional states has given us clues about using odors for weight loss. For example, a number of different studies have demonstrated that when people lose their sense of smell they are at a much higher risk for generalized anxiety disorder.

One theory—not proven yet—is that a kind of free-floating tranquilizing substance (somewhat like a floating valium) is in the air we breath. We refer to such an odor as a subliminal smell because its concentration is just below threshold level, the point at which we can detect it. But just because we don't consciously detect a smell doesn't mean that our brain doesn't know it's there. Subliminal smells are capable of influencing human behavior, and those whose sense of smell is diminished may not benefit from subliminal odors that are part of regulating our moods.

Once we discovered the connection between loss of the ability to smell and anxiety, it was logical to attempt to treat people whose ability to smell is normal but who also have generalized anxiety disorder with odors—assuming that their ability to smell originally fell within the normal range. We're just beginning to explore this concept, but so far the results are encouraging.

For example, we've discovered that inhaling a lavender scent causes changes in brain wave activity in the back of the head, which leads to a more relaxed state. The scent of jasmine, on the other hand, causes changes in the brain waves in the front of the head, which induces a more alert state. In other words, we might use jasmine to help us wake up in the morning and lavender to help us fall asleep at night or to calm our jittery nerves. Early results of our studies indicate that the many millions of people who suffer from insomnia may indeed benefit from inhaling lavender scent before going to bed.

In addition, the results suggest that different forms of anxiety can be treated with a variety of odors, such as apple spice or nutmeg. Patients who were fearful of having an MRI (Magnetic Resonance Imaging) test showed reduced anxiety in the presence of a vanilla scent. The odor of green apple or cucumber sometimes relieves the anxiety that accompanies claustrophobia. Fear or anxiety about a situation leads to generalized frustration—our wants or needs aren't being met at that moment. The odors appear to act on emotional states and help to regulate frustration.

Food odors are valid aids to weight reduction for many reasons. In addition to curtailing appetite or serving as a substitute so as to cut cravings, one additional reason might be that the odors help alleviate frustration, thereby also relieving the need to eat.

We can't always reduce the source of frustration in our lives, but we may be able to use odors to help us cope with them. It's possible that the odors enhance, prolong, or intensify the ability to tolerate the frustration. It's also possible that they switch the focus to something more pleasant. A pleasant odor can trigger associations with a more pleasant time, perhaps even a time in childhood when we were happy and peaceful. The odor can break the cycle of frustration: eating relieves frustration, the person feels bad about eating, these feelings lead to more frustration.

In other words, a significant reason the odors may lead to weight loss is that they help relieve the emotional states that trigger the desire to eat. Just as important, we may form a new habit of reaching for an odor instead of a cookie when tension builds.

Stay Alert and Avoid the Food

Another strategy to prevent overeating involves using odors that keep us in an alert, wakeful state because we are better able to use our intellectual, logical capacities when we are not tired or even drowsy. I once attempted a small weight loss study whose only rule was: no eating after 6:00 P.M. My assumption was that we eat more when we are tired because the rational functions are less dominant. The limbic brain, the seat of our emotional life, tends to dominate when we're tired, which may lead to less-than-rational decisions about food.

Most people who "cheat" on their diets tend to do so during the evening hours. Most people on diets wake up in the morning with great resolve. If they are on a special food plan, they are able to stick to it, usually without significant problems. They may even eat their sensible dinner, just as planned. But their resolve begins to weaken after dinner, when they're relaxing, spending time with the family, or are home alone. The activities that use intellectual capacitates may be over for the day, and fatigue is setting in. The rational brain, the part that says, "Don't eat anymore—you don't need more food," becomes less effective. The message from the limbic brain that says, "That chocolate cake would taste so good—you'll just eat a little piece," begins to become stronger. Some of our study subjects said that the urge to eat during evening hours was *compelling*, nothing like minor temptation that comes and goes or can be pushed away. Before long, the chocolate cake seems like a necessity—at that point, it seems logical to eat the cake. People who are not overweight usually don't understand this. They see food as one of many small temptations and don't comprehend how chocolate cake can come to dominate a person's thoughts.

If you think about it, you can see evidence that behavior is often different during the evening hours. On the negative side, more arguments and even violent fights take place during the evening. Most violent crime is committed at night. People who drink to excess or use other mind-altering drugs tend to gather in groups at night and feel less inhibited about their activities. Most people avoid drinking very much during the day, even at a party. At night, however, their standards may change and they don't understand why they took those last two drinks.

On the positive side, we usually dance or go to movies and seek other forms of entertainment at night, and we tend to reserve the evening for romance and sex. These are all activities that are dominated by the emotional brain. Of course, these events are not by necessity restricted to evening hours, but most societies consider them after-sundown activities because we don't need sharp intellectual functioning to engage in them. As one woman put it, "I read nonfiction during the day, when I can absorb facts, but I read fiction at night, when I want to get involved in a good yarn." Humans are adaptable, and we can learn to be at our intellectual best in the evening if we have to, but it appears that our natural tendency is to think less and feel more at night.

The Brain versus Moral Judgments

It's important to note that brain functions shouldn't be taken lightly or viewed only as a system to manipulate or with which to control behavior. Science has always looked at pathological situations, or the abnormal, to help explain how a normal system works. So it is with the brain.

Some forms of mental retardation—Down's syndrome, for example—are conditions in which the cerebral cortex (the cognitive center of the brain) functions in a limited way. Mentally retarded persons tend to have reduced internal control and may not know when to stop eating. They lack the ability to make that kind of judgment, and unless their diets are carefully monitored, they tend to be overweight. (Many exceptions to this general rule exist, of course.)

On the other hand, in some conditions the limbic functions are so repressed that the cerebral cortex dominates to an abnormal extent. Young women with anorexia nervosa, for example, may believe that their instinctual limbic functions are bad—even evil. Impulses to eat—or to have sex or even to sleep—are viewed as a failure; they signal a failure to control these drives that are signs of weakness. Those with obsessive-compulsive disorders tend to have the same profile. Afraid of their instincts and their emotions, these people struggle to overcome limbic-based impulses.

Small children learn to control their impulses, too, and when they are well-rested, they seem to be good at it. The delightful behavior of a rested toddler is quite a contrast from what happens when he or she is tired. Fatigue "disables" the cerebral cortex, and no situation illustrates this more than one with tired toddlers. They simply can't control themselves when they demand food, but then they throw it on the floor, or they reach for forbidden objects and throw a tantrum when they can't have them. In short, they become wild, and we've all seen it.

Intuitively, we know that fatigue is the root of out-of-control behavior, although that doesn't always make it easier on the parents. The tantrums we see after a stimulating and happy day at an amusement park or a holiday gathering are nothing more than a response to fatigue, a complete inability to control impulses. The limbic brain has taken over, just as it does when that chocolate cake seems like a logical snack to consume at midnight.

Our limbic brain is powerful—it's supposed to be, and we shouldn't condemn it. It is part of a mechanism that helps us survive, and we should avoid condemning it as we struggle to control behavior. Just as a few misguided parents consider a tired child's temper tantrum as evidence that the child is "bad," some people condemn overeating as a sign of moral weakness.

For example, one study participant reported sleepwalking incidents that resulted in taking food out of the refrigerator and eating it, but she wasn't aware of what she'd done until the next morning. She judged herself as morally weak, even though these incidents were just a sign that the primitive brain took charge. Certainly, it was a distressing situation, and she needed help. But she wasn't morally weak.

Much of human behavior is the struggle between the primitive self—Sigmund Freud's id—and the superego, the set of internalized standards or rules that guide what we do. The limbic brain (the id) tells us to eat when the superego (our better judgment) is saying no. One patient described the nighttime urges to eat this way: "It's as if a little person is saying 'I want it, eat that, give it to me now,' and a more rational adult is saying, 'not now—we've had enough food,' and which little guy wins is sometimes up for grabs." Consciously using odors is one way to help the rational brain do its job and quiet the little tantrum thrower. That's why we urge people to keep the odor device handy.

Our study that didn't allow food after 6:00 P.M. was a dismal failure. Why? Because the study subjects couldn't comply. If study subjects can't comply with the guidelines, we might as well abandon the idea—and so we did. To be effective, we must find a way to bypass the compelling messages that have the power to override rational thoughts. The odor devices grew out of our need to find such a tool.

Using odors that keep us alert until we're actually ready to go to bed and sleep is one strategy—not all helpful odors are directly related to food. As mentioned earlier, peppermint and jasmine are examples of stimulating odors. Both odors may act to reduce frustration that is often worse—or seems worse—when we're tired. Everyone would agree that at 2:00 A.M. a problem always seems worse than it is. Odors that keep us alert help enhance the ability of the cerebral cortex to tame or inhibit impulsive drives.

You don't have to use scents in inhalers to benefit from this strategy. Specialty stores sell a variety of scents, including mint and jasmine, in vials that can be used around your home in potpourri mixtures. In time, many more of the stimulating scents will be available in smell devices that look like pens or lipstick containers. The artificial odors work just as well, or in some cases even better than, the scents derived from natural oils. Use room sprays or scented candles as much as you like if you find yourself more wide-awake and alert when you have them around the house. Other strategies include:

- Avoid drinking alcohol before or with your dinner. We know that alcohol inhibits the cerebral cortex, and therefore, the intellectual functions. It's much easier to eat more when the limbic brain dominates. Since it begins to dominate during the evening hours anyway, it makes no sense to further inhibit your rational, logical thought patterns with alcohol.

- If possible, eat dinner no later than 6:00 or 7:00 in the evening. Difficult? No doubt, but you will find it helpful if you can manage it. When the urge to eat begins later in the evening, you now have information that can help you control the impulse rather than condemn it.

One of our patients said that she tells herself that her "thinking brain" is tired and it's allowing her "tantrum brain" to get the upper hand. If she thinks about reaching for ice cream to comfort herself when she's tired, she uses the smell device, and in that short period of time it takes to resist, she thinks of other substitutes—a hot bath or a cup of herb tea, for example. She reminds herself that, by itself, a tempting odor can't control her behavior.

- Exercise early in the day, rather than in the evening. We tend to have increased sense of smell after we exercise vigorously. While many people say they don't feel hungry for several hours after exercising, this isn't universally true. For some people, the heightened ability to smell is enough to tempt them to eat more than they had planned. If they exercise later in the day, they will be more tired and, therefore, more likely to give in to hunger. (More on exercise in the next chapter.)

- Experiment with eating alone and eating with others. Many of us have a tendency to eat more when we eat with other people. However, some people who are trying to lose weight will eat less in the company of other people, perhaps because other emotional needs are being met. When eating alone they eat more because there isn't a signal that tells them the meal is over. Begin to notice which tendency applies to you and try to adjust your meal schedule accordingly. Sometimes we don't have a choice about these things, but self-awareness will help.

- Get plenty of rest. This sounds logical, but in our rushed, stress-packed, and frantic world, millions of people are actually sleep deprived. They don't realize it because they don't suffer from insomnia, and they sleep well—when they finally get around to it. The trouble is, they don't sleep enough. Our best advice is to turn off the television earlier or put down the book before reading just one more chapter. Most people end up fighting to stay awake to jam more activities into the day. This works against sensible eating because more food is consumed in an attempt to stay alert in the evening hours.

To date, we don't have reasons that adequately explain why odors work to reduce frustration and provide an alternative to reaching for our comfort foods. We do know, however, that adding food odors and other scents to our environment helps us cope better with the normal, day-to-day stresses and frustrations we all encounter. If you keep a journal, record how odors affect your ability to break the habit of reaching for food. Like many of our patients, you'll probably be surprised at the insight you gain into your eating patterns.

8 Moving and Losing Weight

During the first year of life, babies are like little Buddhas, with copious fat on their growing bodies. Then, when they become mobile, they generally lose much of that fat as they develop muscle tissue. The more they move—and most babies are unstoppable—the faster new muscle tissue appears. This constant movement develops all types of co-ordination and conditions babies for a lifetime of normal movement.

Much of the excess weight we see among children today can be attributed to a sedentary childhood. In bygone eras, children seldom spent hours inside the house in front of television sets. Most walked to school—and yes, they some-times walked a few miles a day in their round trip. Many worked on farms or in family enterprises, and appetite, food intake, and body weight were usually in a healthy balance.

Unfortunately, we've developed into a society of seden-tary adults, and the children have followed right along. Some dietary changes have no doubt contributed to the shift toward early obesity, but a less mobile lifestyle is probably the bigger factor.

Mobile versus Immobile

What do I mean by mobile? And how have we developed such a sedentary lifestyle? Then too, what does this have to do with exercise—the word many overweight people love to hate? First, no doubt we are more sedentary in our day-to-day lives than ever before and much more immobile than other societies. Since the advent of the automobile, it's not unusual for people to drive one or two blocks to the grocery store rather than walk. This would have been unheard of a generation or two ago. And lest you think I'm blaming the younger people for this trend, let's remember that the older generations started this reliance on the family car—or cars, in many cases.

This move toward immobility, which has affected our children as well as ourselves, has resulted in a proliferation of "artificial" or planned exercise programs. When we walked several blocks to bus stops or spent many hours a week just walking to school or work, plus hauling groceries home, health clubs were usually the designated places for tennis courts and swimming pools, but not aerobics classes, stair-stepping machines, and stationary bikes. Today, however, most people need an additional form of activity beyond the walking they do in the normal course of a day. Cities were once designed for walking and neighborhood shopping, and indeed, some still are. But the design of our current suburbs and small towns is created around shopping malls and four-lane highways. In fact, suburban living as we know it today is possible only because automobiles have eliminated the necessity to work, live, and shop in the same area. Even in many urban areas, public transportation simply augments the car.

And how much walking and general moving around do most people engage in during a typical day? From observing patients and other people—including myself—the automobile and the school bus, not to mention the elevator, have robbed most of us of the very natural tendency to walk from one activity to another.

During the next week, monitor how much moving around you actually do. Do you:

- Drive to work? If so, how far is your workplace? Is it possible for you walk if you allowed extra time every day? (There isn't a right or wrong answer here. I'm not suggesting that you change your lifestyle all at once—and I don't think you can simply move within walking distance of your office just because it used to be commonplace.)

- Climb stairs? If you work on a second or third floor of an office building, do you take the elevator or climb the stairs? If you take the elevator, why? Have you tried climbing a flight or two of stairs? If you have stairs in your home, do you try to save trips up and down the stairs rather than considering the activity as normal exercise?

- Walk to the supermarket or convenience store? Do you know how far it is? If your car breaks down, how would you bring food into your home?

- Move around your home? Do you garden? Do you stand up while you cook or work on a project in your basement? Do you carry laundry up or down stairs? When you come home from work, what is your lifestyle like? Are you sedentary—the proverbial couch potato?

- When was the last time you took a walk after dinner? What is stopping you from doing so?

- And do you engage in a form of recreational exercise with regularity? By group exercise I mean tennis, a hiking or cycling club, racquetball, a softball team, volleyball at the neighborhood park, and so forth. (If you're wondering why I didn't put golf on this list, I'd have to say that driving around in carts is hardly what I'd call exercise. If you like golf, by all means, keep playing, but try to avoid using a cart, or you can't count on it to help you to lose or maintain weight.)

If you're like most overweight people, your weekly move-ment inventory probably resembles Joanie's, one of our study subjects. After she had lost some weight, she asked about losing pounds more quickly and most important, keeping the unwanted weight off. When asked about ex-ercise, she said: "I hate exercise—I get tired after two minutes and feel so discouraged that I can't bring myself to go to the gym. Besides, I'm embarrassed there—all those slim, young bodies make me feel just that much older and flabbier."

This is such a common response that I prefer to start a discussion of exercise by talking about moving. If you've just started the using-odors-for-weight-loss program, you might have a low opinion of formal exercise programs, too. If so, for the first weeks or even months of the program, concen-trate on using the odors, making them a new habit. And, as an additional motivator and to help you feel better physi-cally and mentally, think about how much you move around.

When we talked with Joanie, we suggested that she start by climbing the stairs to her third-floor office. Even walking *down* the stairs is an improvement on no movement at all, which perfectly described her lifestyle. Next, think about walking to the nearest store rather than jumping in the car. Joanie was four blocks from the grocery store. She lived with her teenage son, and she was used to buying large quantities of groceries at one time. But, as a way to force herself to move, she began walking the four blocks—eight blocks round trip—and sent her son for heavy items that she couldn't carry. (He balked, to be sure. He was used to being chauffeured almost everywhere, and he didn't like this new "walking bit," as he called it. He too, however, had a ten-dency to overeat and gain weight. He was fighting both a genetic tendency and a sedentary lifestyle, and she was helping him in the long run by coaxing him to move.)

As a teenager, Joanie played volleyball and she liked to swim, but as an overweight adult, she had given up not just organized activity, but any activity at all. In other words, she'd become a slave to the car, always parking it in a spot closest to her destination. In fact, her life had revolved around ways to limit her physical activity because she was so uncomfortable, both physically and in a social sense. It had taken her years to develop this pattern, and it wasn't going to change overnight.

You Don't Have to Start with Vigorous Aerobics or Jogging

When people haven't exercised at all, forcing them into health club aerobics classes or onto treadmills is often futile. Along with the failed diet, the exercise program fails too. For this reason, I helped Joanie and others ease into exercise by encouraging them to move around—walk instead of ride, climb stairs instead of taking elevators, stand up while they cook, dig in the garden, and so forth. In other words, I encourage movement in whatever form it takes.

This is not to say that I actually discourage people from starting regular exercise programs, *after checking with their family physicians, of course*. Indeed, many study subjects engaged in some exercise, and I encouraged them to increase the frequency and length of workout sessions as the pounds began to come off.

My primary concern, however, is to promote success in losing weight and keeping it off. I want you to learn new habits over time, not all at once. The odor devices will help you lose pounds and form new habits, beginning with eating less food at each meal. Walking up some stairs and leaving the car behind when your destination is a few blocks away is another way to begin a new habit—the habit of moving.

Let me put my opinion another way. If I told you that the program described in this book included a certain amount and kind of exercise and restrictions on the kind of food you eat every day, you would probably get that familiar sinking feeling. You might think that this is just another book that's filled with instructions about what you *should* do, what you *can't* do, what you have to *change*, and on and on. Most of our study subjects had been through years of this kind of "advice." They'd had it with these programs and diets and couldn't listen anymore. Besides, as Joanie said, "It's not as if I live in a glass bubble—I already knew much of what the diet people told me—I couldn't do it, but I was aware."

Okay, I'll Start Moving—But What Then?

Joanie began moving around more; it was a moderate change in her lifestyle. She had lost 7 pounds during the first month of the odor program, and she was feeling better. For about six additional weeks, she limited her exercise to the increased walking she did a few times a week and the stairs she climbed. But she also found herself more active in small ways. She scraped and painted the walls of her bedroom, cleaned out a few closets, and started walking to her church, which was about five blocks from her home. Each bit of activity added to her sense of accomplishment, and before long, she was ready to try something she'd once dreaded.

One day while Joanie was in the video store renting a movie, she saw an exercise tape that promised it was designed for many levels of exercise proficiency—no difficult dance steps, no jumping around, and so forth. She bought it, with only slight guilt over the fact that years before, she'd given a library of exercise videos to the church rummage sale. "They were all so difficult for an overweight person to do," she said, "that I became discouraged and decided to get rid of them. Now, here I was starting again. I couldn't help but wonder if I was throwing away more money."

I believe that home exercise videos are a wonderful innovation for people who can't get to health clubs on a regular basis or don't want to exercise with others. Nowadays, the wide variety of tapes available means that you *can* find some to meet your needs. Many feature low-impact aerobics, and some are designed for people just starting out. In the privacy of her own home, Joanie could work at her own pace. At first, she ended up marching in place for much of the video because she couldn't keep up, and so, she bought another tape that was even more basic. Eventually, she had a variety of videos, and within a few months, she was doing some beginning step aerobics. She made it her goal to do the exercise three to four times a week, which began to speed up her weight loss.

So, Do I Have to Do Aerobics?

Joanie's solution to the exercise dilemma was to walk more, move more, and use aerobic videotapes. Many mothers of small children find that they couldn't exercise at all if it weren't for videotapes. This solution works for them. But John's solution was much different. He lived near a state park that had walking trails, and he began walking for thirty to forty-five minutes five days a week. He also lived in the Southeast, where he rarely had to cancel his walk because of cold weather, and the walking became a good exercise for him. You see, John had a sedentary job, and he had to drive forty minutes each way. Two restaurants were adjacent to his office building, and opportunities to move around on his job or during lunch hour were almost nonexistent. His wife was a regular walker, and he started going with her. She was happy for the company, and he was getting badly needed exercise.

Probably the most popular forms of exercise today are brisk walking, jogging, the stationary cycle, and aerobic exercise in the form of videos or classes. All are what we call fat-burning exercise. This means that they raise the heart rate and keep it raised over a sustained period of time, providing a cardiovascular workout, meaning that these exercises condition the heart.

Just because I don't attempt the impossible and demand that you exercise, that doesn't mean I don't urge you to begin moving and adopt some form of physical exercise that provides cardiovascular conditioning. Heart disease is the number one cause of death in our country, and while many factors place us at risk, obesity and a sedentary lifestyle are two major ones. People whose weight is normal are still urged to exercise for a healthy heart.

Aren't Some Forms of Exercise Dangerous?

I'm not asking you to take up rock climbing or white-water rafting—for the unskilled, these are dangerous activities. But for the most part, exercise programs that start slowly and build fitness and endurance over time are not dangerous. You should always check with your doctor before you begin any exercise program. Most people, however, are able to walk a few blocks just to begin the habit of moving around and can do so without any concern at all.

I can almost guarantee that your doctor will stand up and cheer if you ask him or her if it's okay if you start walking thirty to sixty minutes a few times a week. And the reaction is likely to be the same if you start working out on an exercise bicycle or with a tape. Chances are you've been urged to do so anyway. The key is to start slowly—I'm quite sure your doctor will agree.

Many books are available about target heart rates and optimal length of exercise sessions and so forth. You can even find estimates of how many calories are burned during an hour of walking versus forty-five minutes of rowing and jogging versus cycling. I'm not as concerned about the number of calories burned as I am about fitting regular exercise into a normal lifestyle and doing it safely. You are exercising safely if:

- you can talk to another person briefly while you are working out, without gasping for air.

- you are breathing deeply, but never fighting for air.

- you don't have pain in your knees and ankles (some stiffness is bound to appear when you first start, but you should never experience severe pain).

- you are energized rather than exhausted—you're overdoing it for your fitness level if you collapse on the couch and need a nap after a workout. Exercise gives us energy because it sends oxygen to every cell in our body. It wakes up a sluggish system; it should not cause fatigue.

- you find that you have more upbeat and cheerful moods—an improved sense of general well-being. Exercise affects brain chemistry and encourages the production of endorphins, chemicals in the brain that promote mental well-being and are also the body's natural pain killers. You've probably heard of the "runner's high," and that phenomenon is real for many people. Increased endorphin production is the key to that mental state.

Doesn't Exercise Affect My Metabolism— And Won't This Alter the Set Point?

It's long been known that regular exercise promotes weight loss and helps maintain normal weight. You don't see overweight track and field athletes, marathon runners, and so forth, precisely because those activities boost metabolism and build muscle tissue. Your metabolism is the rate at which your body burns fuel—the calories consumed in food. People who exercise regularly are often able to eat more because they are efficiently burning the calories they take in.

Exercise speeds up metabolic rate, provided it is done over a sustained period of time—about thirty minutes or more. In addition, the revved-up metabolic rate lasts for several hours after the exercise session. For this reason, I encourage people to exercise energetically, but not to be too concerned with the number of calories they're burning. The post-exercise metabolic boost isn't easy to calculate, but realize that it's there.

In addition, exercise builds muscle tissue, which uses more calories to maintain than fat tissue. In other words, the more muscle mass you have, the more fuel you burn, which makes it easier for physically fit people to stay slimmer and fit. It's easier because they can eat more food without gaining weight.

Exercise is the one known way to alter the body's set point, the weight the body considers normal and will fight to maintain. The metabolic change coupled with increased muscle tissue are the keys to altering set point. As we've said, the body will fight for homeostasis—it is designed that way to protect us. If we starve ourselves and move around less, the body will adjust the metabolism to hoard body fat. When we exercise and eat normally (but in smaller quantities), the increased metabolic rate readjusts the set point.

Undoubtedly, exercise is your friend in losing weight and maintaining lost pounds. It might not seem like it right now, but after you begin losing weight by using the odors, you'll feel better and begin moving around more—just parking father away from the mall entrance is a start—and you'll want to add some regular exercise into your life.

You Don't Have to Do This Alone

Most of our study subjects were not interested in health club exercise programs—at least at first. But that doesn't mean that they didn't want or need moral support. In the last few years, I've noticed groups of people out walking, jogging, or cycling together. In fact, walking clubs and groups are common now, and in some towns, the local malls have opened their doors to walkers before shopping hours, sometimes in cooperation with heart fitness programs sponsored by local hospitals. If such a program interests you, call your local hospital or mall and find out about its walking program.

Cindy and Alice, our smell buddies, were not able to exercise together very often, but they checked in with each other and gave support. About twice a month, they took a long walk in a nearby forest preserve with their children. Both said they would not have been motivated to do this alone—they needed each other's company. Their walks also added variety to their exercise program.

Cindy was able to find two neighborhood women to walk with on Saturday mornings and one evening during the week. Groups of neighbors walking and jogging together is so commonplace now that I'm beginning to think it's a trend—and one worth promoting. In fact, I wonder if the emphasis on exercise that is so pervasive today isn't improving communities by encouraging people to be outside exploring their neighborhoods and meeting other people. Cindy told us that she hadn't known her neighbor's name, but she passed her house every Saturday morning. It was on one of those walks that the neighbor came out and asked her if she'd mind some company. A walking partnership was formed.

Some people become more motivated if they exercise in facilities such as parks, the YMCA or YWCA, or health clubs. Some people consider it a needed break from their homes and all the demands that await there. Some companies have access to discounts on health club memberships, so check that out if you decide you'd like company and support from other people. If you're going to join a club, be sure it is open seven days a week for long hours, so that scheduling isn't an issue.

Variety Is the Spice

We often think of an exercise program as one activity that we favor above all others. If you want to run marathons eventually, as Oprah Winfrey did, then you will probably need to start with walking, move to jogging, and train for the event. (Ms. Winfrey has spoken publicly, not only about her lifelong struggle with weight but also about learning to enjoy exercise and accepting that it must be part of her life if she is to maintain a normal weight. In this role, she has become a valuable public educator.) However, you might not have that ambition, and nothing is wrong with that. It isn't necessary for you to choose between walking or cycling or doing an exercise tape. In fact, varying your routine may be the very thing you need in order to stick to a program.

Lisa dusted off the exercise bicycle, dragged it out of the basement, and put it in a corner of the bedroom, where she'd be reminded to use it once a week. Her husband complained, though, and told her that if she was using it only once a week, he didn't see the point. Wasn't it just taking up space? But her once-a-week bike ride was augmented with a twice-weekly walk with a friend and using an exercise video—the step-aerobics variety—at least once a week. Doing the same activity over and over bored her. She knew she would find excuses not to exercise if she couldn't add some variety.

If you have the need to beat the boredom of one or even two activities, consider the following:

- Yoga—a perfect exercise to promote flexibility, balance, and posture. It also prevents back and joint problems and is regularly recommended as a rehabilitative exercise for people recovering from musculoskeletal injuries. Of course, I realize that yoga is associated with the religious schools and traditions of Hinduism, and it is used as part of spiritual training for millions of people. However, *hatha* yoga, the level of yoga that emphasizes physical movements and postures, is available in the West, and nowadays yoga classes are common in even very small communities. Many people find that the physical benefits of yoga eventually take second place to the mental benefits, which include quieting the mind, increased concentration, and deep relaxation. Even people suffering with arthritis can benefit from yoga.

• T'ai Chi—performed as a series of movements, T'ai Chi comes to us from China and also has a spiritual component. However, its movements emphasize flexibility and strength and, therefore, may be of great benefit to those who need exercise that moves all the muscle groups without undo strain. T'ai Chi is a discipline, and like yoga, it has mental benefits as well as physical. I have known people who have come to believe that T'ai Chi has added to their quality of life, physically and mentally. (This is the idea with both yoga and T'ai Chi—they were never developed nor designed as only exercise programs. Most people consider them pathways to the meditative state.)

• Toning exercises and weight training—for the most part, toning can be done with an exercise video, and many are available in stores and catalogs. Health clubs also offer toning classes. Weight training is best learned from an experienced person, and almost every health club has a weight trainer on staff. Both toning and weight training are excellent exercise programs to help people become strong and fit as they lose weight. As we said, muscle tissue uses more fuel than fat tissue, so converting fat into muscle will help you keep your momentum and will fight against plateaus—those frustrating periods when the scale doesn't want to budge.

These are only suggestions—don't limit yourself to them. Once you know it is safe for you to exercise, then engage in any activity that appeals to you. Start slowly—or, I should say, train slowly. You can't whip a body into shape, but you can ease it in the right direction.

What about Odors and Exercise?

Much of the work we do at our foundation involves re-searching the effects of odors, both good and bad, on human behavior in a number of arenas, from learning to buying habits. Several studies have established that bad odors can make people more aggressive, and we once tested this theory on male athletes. We found that in the presence of a bad smell, these participants exercised harder—more vigorously—and they burned calories at a faster rate than athletes who were performing their exercise without the addition of an unpleasant odor.

Now don't be alarmed. I'm not suggesting that you make your house smell foul in order to burn a few more calories during a session on the treadmill. That's taking the phrase "no pain, no gain" entirely too far. Aversion therapy doesn't work because people won't use it, and no one would pay good money to go to a health club that smells bad— I wouldn't either. However, our results prompted us to examine exercise patterns in the presence of pleasant odors—those scents that most people like.

Popcorn and strawberry are generally thought to be pleasant odors, and just as with the bad smell, the men in our study burned more calories and exercised harder in the presence of either odor.(The study subjects wore masks that were infused with the odor.) We aren't sure why this is so, but we know that pleasant odors appear to help people exercise longer and more vigorously. For example, the scent might serve as a distraction, much the way watching tele-vision while walking on a treadmill is a distraction. It's also possible that the odors lifted mood, and when people feel better, they exercise harder and longer because they don't tire as easily.

I can't tell you that you will lose weight faster if you use an odor in your home while you exercise. The research is too new, and we don't have conclusive results about specific odors. (Strawberry and popcorn worked, but lavender or cheese pizza might have worked too. More research is needed.) However, I encourage you to try odors for yourself. Burn a scented candle or spray the room with your favorite room spray. The most important benefit is that you are creating a pleasant environment, one that lifts your mood and perhaps makes it easier to slip the tape into the VCR. Eventually, more research will probably isolate certain odors, and I predict that one day a commercial product will be designed that infuses the room with a scent that keeps you on the exercise bicycle just a bit longer.

In Summary

- Get your doctor's advice before you change your exercise patterns. Find out what if any limits you have. I want you to begin putting your body in motion, but I also want you to be safe.

- Move around in small ways—walk instead of ride, park farther away from the door, walk up and down the stairs, move around your office and home as much as possible. Encourage your children to do the same.

- Schedule your exercise—don't leave it to chance. Engaging in some physical activity every day is terrific, but if you can do it only three or four times a week, that's good too.

- Don't compete with anyone else. If you haven't walked in years, go at your own pace and don't worry about others passing you by. If you're in an aerobics class, then do only as much as you can without gasping for air. But keep moving, even if you only walk in place. In a few weeks, you'll see real progress. If you are pressured to do more, talk with the instructor and explain your situation. You risk injury if you do too much all at once.

- Add variety to your exercise plans. There is no reason for you to be bored with exercise—you have too many choices. There is no one right exercise program. If you are stiff and want to add flexibility, toning, and muscle strength, then try yoga or T'ai Chi or find a weight trainer who can work with you on flexibility.

- Think in terms of thirty-minute aerobic exercise blocks. You can exercise longer, but if you sustain an activity for thirty minutes, you are getting the cardio-vascular benefits. Your other movement activity— short walks, climbing stairs, and so forth—are good for you and should help get you started, but over time, you'll find you feel better and lose weight faster with regular, sustained periods of activity.

- Remember that exercise isn't a substitute for using the odors. Exercise is a habit you can form right along with losing weight with odors.

9 Filling Your Plate

If you did nothing more than use the odor devices frequently every day, you would probably begin dropping unwanted pounds because you would consume less food. Our study clearly showed that weight loss is possible without a required food plan and a list of forbidden foods. The rate of your weight loss would vary, depending on many factors, including the number of times you're sniffing the inhaler, the size and frequency of your meals, the amount and quality of your exercise, and so forth.

Our study subjects began losing weight because they began leaving food on their plates and, in general, were eating smaller portions. For the most part, they were able to eat with the family at home, have meals in restaurants, or have lunch with their colleagues. They lived a regular, normal life, however they defined it.

That said, I would be remiss as a physician if I didn't discuss some basic components of a healthful diet. However, I want you to discuss guidelines for healthful eating with your family physician. If you are on a special diet and have dietary restrictions, then by all means continue following the medical advice you've been given. Nothing I've said in this book is meant to be a substitute for medical care or advice.

A Healthful Diet Isn't What It Used to Be

If it seems that dietary guidelines have changed, you're right. For many years, dairy and meat products were emphasized in the American diets, while today, they are still included, but in smaller amounts. For the most part, the changes have come because excess fat intake—the high-fat diet—is associated with higher risk of developing heart disease and even some cancers. High-fat intake is also associated with obesity, which itself is a risk factor for many diseases, including, of course, heart disease, hypertension, diabetes, and stroke.

Back in the fifties and continuing through the seventies, schoolchildren were taught that they must have two servings of dairy and two servings of meat every day to be healthy. The cereal and bread and the fruit and vegetable groups were represented, too, with four servings recommended from each group. These were minimums, and beyond these guidelines we could fill our diets with whatever food items we chose.

Times changed, however, and in 1992, the U.S. Department of Agriculture issued new dietary guidelines, which rearranged the food groups into a pyramid emphasizing what are known as complex carbohydrates—whole grains, legumes (lentils and split peas, for example), and beans—with eleven servings a day recommended. Three other food groups are built from the wide base of complex carbohydrates, and in ascending order, they are: vegetables (three to five daily servings) and fruit (two to four daily servings); dairy, meat, chicken, and fish (two to three daily servings from dairy and the same from the animal protein group); and fats and sweets, which sit at the very tip of the pyramid, not because they are more important but because the tip of a pyramid is the smallest section. This is no accident. Reducing fat intake is the primary goal of these new dietary guidelines, and increased fiber intake is the other significant goal of the diet represented by the food pyramid.

It has been said that the percentages allotted to each category of food closely resemble the typical Asian diet and also that of the Mediterranean countries. (In both regions, incidence of heart disease is significantly lower than it is in Northern Europe and the United States, although other factors contribute to the risk, including genetics.) Obviously, vegetarians consume most of their protein from grains and beans and dairy products, although some vegetarians do not eat animal-based protein in any form, including milk.

The advent of the food pyramid has been good news in most ways. Americans are rethinking their emphasis on meat at every meal, and more people are eating whole grains and more fresh vegetables—or at least they're conscious of the need to eat this way. From what I see, not only among my patients, but also from simple observation, many people are having difficulty figuring out how to consume less fat and shift their diets to meet the new guidelines.

What Did Our Study Tell Us?

Telling overweight people to eat controlled portions of one food or another is often the cause of rampant "diet failure" in the first place. To me, the biggest risk factor our study subjects shared was being overweight. The purpose of the study was to see if odors could assist people in their weight loss efforts. We believed we could discuss dietary issues, such as lowering fat and increasing fiber, with our participants when they began feeling better emotionally and physically. Then, too, we knew that when it came time to talk about maintaining weight loss, our study subjects would likely have the mental attitude needed to pay attention to our advice. In other words, attempting too many changes all at once is usually self-defeating.

So, what happened during the first weeks and months of our study? As we've said, the odors helped participants eat less. But, eat less of what? Well, many people were used to eating fast food. One woman said that she still ordered her typical Whopper or Big Mac, but she consumed about half of it. Was this low fat? Not exactly, but this woman consumed less fat at each meal without counting fat grams. Certainly, eating less of a high-fat diet is not optimal, but she was taking on what she could handle at that time—and her slimmer figure encouraged her to keep going.

One of the men in our study named pizza as his favorite food. He and his office partner had a pizza delivered for their lunch almost every day. Most of the time, they ate the whole thing. But, by using the inhaler, he found that he ate one or two pieces and saved the rest for dinner or the next day. We didn't tell him to eat a low-fat diet, but he consumed less fat, nonetheless.

Our participants' experiences confirmed my thinking that a prescribed diet wouldn't have worked well with our approach. Kim, a woman who had well over 100 pounds to lose, talked to us about the numerous rebounds she'd experienced over a period of about twenty years. Deprivation caused her to go off a low-fat, "sensible" diet and consume great quantities of food, often the refined carbohydrates found in typical baked goods. When she marshaled her courage, she went back to counting calories, weighing and measuring, counting fat grams, and all the rest of the routines she'd become accustomed to. The cycle had continued for years.

Kim is a success story in that she found, for the first time in her life, that she could eat less of what she called "regular" food and drop weight slowly. People like Kim know the drill, so to speak. Experienced dieters don't need me to tell them that baked skinless chicken breasts have less fat than fried chicken wings, skin and all. They don't necessarily need to be told that lean ground sirloin has less fat per serving than pepperoni pizza. However, it's a big relief to begin using odors and concentrate just on them, rather than being conscious all the time of calorie and fat intake.

In terms of long-term weight loss, I'd much rather see a person use an odor device, sniff away, and lose some weight, without herculean efforts to avoid certain foods. Eating half a dessert once in a while does not mean that one has "blown" this program. In fact, many of our patients never changed their diets at all.

It's no wonder dieters are confused when they once were told to avoid baked potatoes and pasta like the plague— one woman even called these foods "fat foods," and foods like baked fish, "skinny foods." Now they are told to limit protein and eat potatoes and pasta. If you like pasta, I'd go ahead and eat it as long as you use the odors to help you limit your portions and stop eating before you've consumed the whole plate. Restaurant portions of foods such as pasta tend to be far larger than they need to be, and taking half the plate home to eat the next day is probably a sensible goal.

So, Is Eating Less Fat Important in the Long Run?

Eating less fat than the typical American diet provides is important—any dietician or physician will tell you that. But that is not the same as eliminating fat from the diet. We need fat for many physiological functions, including hormone production. A diet too low in fat can be very dangerous. Fats are not created equal, however. The type of fat that we are generally advised to limit is saturated fat—butter, margarine, and other solid vegetable fats—and the animal fats found in red meat, whole milk, and so forth. We are encouraged to get the fat we need from unsaturated fats, such as canola, sesame, olive oils.

We are fortunate in that the issue of reducing fat in the diet is the focus of many health and general interest magazines, cookbooks, the cooking shows on television, and many restaurants. There are even food magazines that specialize just in low-fat cooking. Many restaurants provide nutrition breakdowns of selected menu items. You can order a dish and know how many total calories are in it, plus get a count of fat, carbohydrate, and protein grams. New food labeling laws also help, and many patients have commented that they appreciate being warned about the high fat content of many prepared foods, from frozen entrées to packaged desserts.

Because so much information is available about low-fat eating and your own physician can steer you in the right direction, I won't belabor the issue here. However, I'm still concerned about deprivation and the long-term effects of severely restricted eating. I prefer that people think about ways to make dietary adjustments slowly (unless their physicians have advised them to make bigger changes right away) so that a new way of eating can become permanent.

Oprah Winfrey again provides a good example of changes that didn't turn her life upside down, but that worked nonetheless. After attempting a number of different diets, Ms. Winfrey finally announced that she would never diet again. She had been through all the stages of hope and disappointment and faced the fact that she needed to find a different way of eating, one that took the focus off the numbers on the scale. A couple of years later, Rosie Daley, Ms. Winfrey's personal chef, published a cookbook, *In the Kitchen with Rosie,* which includes reduced-fat recipes that Rosie Daley developed.

The cookbook amazes many dieters. How could sweet potato pie or oatmeal muffins be "diet" food? Or how about french fries and pizza? Yet, the book contains recipes for dishes that anyone would consider gourmet food. Ms. Winfrey couldn't believe it herself. In her introduction to the book, she talks about once believing that healthful eating meant feeling deprived, but once she understood that low-fat, low-sugar, and low-salt food could be delicious and emotionally satisfying, she changed her relationship with food forever.

This is the kind of dietary change I admire and would like to see you try, too. Ms. Winfrey's role as a talk-show host has influenced many issues in our country. But I consider one of her most important contributions to be her willingness to discuss her struggle with being overweight and passing on information about how she stabilized her weight by learning a new way of eating. And, of course, as I've said, she exercises, too, and realizes that activity must be part of her lifestyle no matter what other demands on her time she faces.

Rather than giving up all her favorite foods, Ms. Winfrey ate slightly different versions of them, lost weight, and developed a more healthy attitude toward weight control. I advise my patients to do the same. Eat smaller portions of food you enjoy, facilitated by the odor inhalers, and learn new ways to prepare your favorite foods. With all the "healthy heart" cookbooks available to us nowadays, this isn't difficult to do. And you never need to count calories again.

Leaving the Table

Using odors to lose weight, without adding a food plan or diet, seems odd to many people, perhaps because our approach starts with questions about why we feel full rather than why we feel hungry. We attempt to help people stop eating as much food as they might be used to, and the odors are the primary tool we use.

However, the question about why anyone stops eating is an open one. We know that feeling full doesn't necessarily make us leave the table. In fact, we've all had the experience of eating until we are uncomfortable at holiday dinners or other celebrations. And we know that eating doesn't stop because blood sugar is back to a normal level. As we've noted, unless you have diabetes or reactive hypoglycemia, your blood sugar at the beginning of a meal is about the same as it is at the end.

As it turns out, many reasons cause us to stop eating at any point. As you continue using the inhalers and are eating less, consider all the reasons you stop consuming a meal or a snack. Notice your own behavior and that of others.

Some people stop eating when all the food on their plate is gone. They don't necessarily think about second helpings. Those who do fill their plates a second time eat every last bite of that food, too. When I was young, I was told to leave a bit of food on the plate—that was part of good table manners. Other people, however, were told that cleaning the plate was a sign of good manners and leaving food was terribly rude.

Many of our study participants were raised to believe that leaving food on the plate was wasteful and insulting to the cook. Therefore, they were obligated to eat every scrap. Leaving half a Big Mac behind was a new experience; some said they felt guilty because others in the world were starving. One man said, "It's taken me a lifetime to get over the idea that I must eat what's on my plate because some people don't have enough to eat. Throwing away food was considered a sin my household. I finally figured out that my extra hundred pounds isn't helping hungry people and it's hurting me. This is logical, of course, but old habits and messages around food die hard."

Most people who sincerely want to control their weight will eventually understand that they are not obligated to consume food just because it's in front of them—and because someone, down the block or thousands of miles away, lacks sufficient food. We can find plenty of valid ways to address the issue of widespread hunger and malnutrition, but overeating ourselves isn't one of them.

Other people were urged to eat so that there would be

no leftovers. A woman told us about her severely over-weight mother, who ate the portions of food left over in the serving dishes and pots and pans. "She was a human garbage disposal, and when I was first married I started the same pattern. I'm just glad I am able to see that sometimes, excess food is better off in the garbage than piling up around my waistline." This is not an uncommon experience. But we don't need to keep repeating these patterns. We can stop eating when we leave the table and, if not enough food is left for another meal, scrape it into the garbage. It's that simple.

Sometimes we stop eating for social reasons. Others at the table have put their forks down, so we do, too. Or we look at the clock and see it's time to get back to work. We may leave food behind because we're obligated to be some-where else. Some people say they stop eating when the waistline on their pants or skirt is tight.

There are many reasons we stop eating, including of course, that we feel full. The odors appear to trigger the satiety center to signal a sense of fullness, that when put in words means, "You've had enough food for now. Leave the table." Many people, however, find it helpful to examine all the other reasons they stop eating. Awareness of old patterns can be especially helpful if pushing the chair away from the table has been difficult.

Keeping It Simple

For now, I reiterate my theory that deprivation is the enemy of persons who desire weight loss. To begin losing weight, just start using the odors and eat regular meals. Keep sniffing the odors and watch the amount of food you eat shrink. Take smaller helpings and resist filling the plate again—the odors will help you. As you begin losing weight, start thinking about ways you can make your favorite dishes with less salt, sugar, and fat. Then take a look at the reduced fat and salt items on the menus of your favorite restaurants.

If you've been used to plain food, try different kinds of food. If you keep using the odor devices, you'll feel free to eat a wide variety of ethnic foods, from Thai to Guatemalan, but you won't overeat because the odors help you know when to stop.

And please, don't be hard on yourself because a rich dessert looks good to you. These treats probably always will have appeal, and unless you have specific health concerns, there is no reason you can't enjoy them now and then, especially if you exercise regularly.

"Lite" Can Be Deceptive

The new food labeling guidelines help us assess fat gram and calorie content of our food. This is fine, and I encourage you to read labels and compare products. What you will probably see, however, is that "reduced fat," or "low salt," or "sugar-free" doesn't necessarily mean low calorie. As I said in chapter 4, artificial sweeteners can actually cause hunger, meaning that artificially sweetened food that's advertised as a dieter's friend may be the dieter's enemy instead.

There is a sensible way to eat "lite," but many people misinterpret a statement such as "fat-free." As patients have said, "It's as easy to overeat the low-fat, sugar-free foods as it is to overeat the regular variety." The key to making the most of "lite" foods is to eat less of them, certainly no more than you would eat of the regular variety. I would also avoid the artificially sweetened foods, unless your doctor has advised you to use them. (Diabetics, for example, are some-times steered to artificially sweetened products.) The odors will help you limit your portions, which is the most reliable way to get rid of excess pounds.

10 *Why Do Odors Work?*

We know from our research results that people can lose weight with odors—that's clear. If you begin using odors and your unwanted pounds start to disappear, you, like many other people, will become even more curious about the mechanism of the weight loss you're experiencing. Of course, this discussion may not interest you, and if that's the case, I recommend that you skip it. Just use the other information in the book and watch excess weight disappear. For some people, just knowing that the odors work for them is enough. They don't care about the how or the why of the program.

However, many individuals, who are also delighted with their results, have an intellectual curiosity about the mechanism and become eager to learn more about odors and the way they affect human behavior in many areas of life, not just in weight control. There are a number of possible mechanisms, and as research continues, we'll probably be able to define them more clearly. We've already discussed some of them throughout this book. For example, we talked about odors that keep us alert and help tame the little id, who is concerned only about basic drives and doesn't care that we weigh too much. We also discussed the idea that odors can help us overcome cravings.

Because odors affect human behavior in so many ways, it is difficult to isolate one mechanism and say "that's it, we've unlocked the secret door." In truth, it's entirely possible that the whole array of mechanisms, from fooling the satiety center to changing a habit, play a role in odors and weight control. In other words, the explanations given here are not meant as either/or possibilities. Right now, we prefer to think of them as both/and, inclusive, and perhaps working in tandem. One day we might discover that all the explanations are correct, meaning that these different responses interact with each other.

Responses might also be individual. Perhaps one set of mechanisms dominates in one person and a different set in another. Or the mechanisms might change in the same person throughout the day.

First, as we've discussed, the odors have a direct effect on the satiety center, localized in a specific area, the ventromedial nucleus of the hypothalamus, which is the master gland of the body. The established connection between odors and the satiety center is certainly one of the reasons we began to explore the relationship between odors and weight control. As described earlier, we know that if the satiety center is damaged in a guinea pig, it will literally eat until it dies.

You will notice that as you use the odors more, you will reach for food less. This is the reason we asked people to estimate how often they use the devices and noted that the more they sniffed, the faster they lost. It's as if the satiety center was constantly stimulated, and hunger became less of an issue. From airline pilots (some of whom have trouble staying out of the snack food during long, usually dull flights) to school teachers who experience daylong stress to office workers whose coworkers bring a different "treat" in every day, more sniffing meant more lost pounds.

Going to the Dogs

A second possible mechanism is related to deconditioning the Pavlovian conditioned response to food. The Russian physiologist Ivan Pavlov trained dogs to salivate at the sound of a bell and conditioned the dogs to associate the sound of the bell with the sight of food. Although he later won the Nobel Prize for far greater accomplishments, he is best remembered for his dog experiments. In fact, the expression "just like Pavlov's dogs" is part of our popular culture, and virtually everyone knows that it refers to a conditioned response. In the popular sense, we associate the expression with any conditioned response, such as stopping at a red light or stop sign. We automatically hit the brake because we're conditioned to.

The Pavlovian joke is on us, of course, because humans smell food, begin to salivate, and become hungry. It's just as conditioned in us as it is in dogs. Pavlov's experiments were actually conducted because he was studying digestion, not because he wanted to study human conditioned response behavior.

It's possible that these odor devices work for weight control because they are food smells, and if you detect a food odor in the absence of actual food, the reflex response will change. If you use the inhalers often, you'll eventually break the connection between a food odor and real food. Over time, you can be around food and food odors and not feel the compulsion to eat. In a sense, we're fooling the brain and breaking a conditioned response at the same time.

If It's Not One Thing, It's Another

If you've been using the inhalers, you've no doubt noticed that the urge for a chocolate bar or a doughnut is displaced by the odor. You're essentially changing a behavior by displacing, or substituting, it with another behavior. A smoker might displace the urge to smoke by chewing gum; a nail-biter might displace the urge to nibble on her nails by applying nail polish.

Some of our study participants became conscious of the inhaler as a displacement mechanism in that they made the connection between an urge to eat and a substitute behavior. Some said they grabbed their journal as well as the inhaler, and the desire to eat a cookie out of the box that was being passed around the office went away—usually quite quickly. The act of writing a sentence or two in the journal immediately after sniffing the odor was enough to get them past a powerful urge.

And let's be clear again about something. An urge to eat may be powerful, but it isn't "bad." Seasoned dieters (and others who believe they must be in perfect control every minute) are so used to associating giving in to temptation with being bad that they are often very hard on themselves. They believe that if eating a piece of candy is "bad" for their diets, then they must be bad people. In our culture, temptation is often seen as the same as actually carrying out the action. Hence, a dieter is tempted and feels like a failure.

Displacement is not a sign of weakness, which is important to remember if you start feeling foolish about substituting one behavior with another. One woman said, "I feel like a child. Shouldn't I be adult enough to just say no to desserts and junk food?" But this isn't a matter of being a "grown-up." The urge to eat when food is available is an important physiological response, linked to our evolutionary past. Without it, we probably wouldn't have survived. Besides, we're always displacing one behavior with another any time we want to change a habit or a pattern. We need to stop making moral judgments about cravings or temptations; just substitute the inhaler for a while and let the self-chastising behavior go.

Don't Forget, You Don't Have to Eat That Right Now

Another important mechanism of the odor device is that it acts as a concrete reminder that you really don't want to eat.

Perhaps you've taped a picture of a thin person on the refrigerator—women tend to do this more than men. I've spoken with many women who were motivated, at least for a while, because they often chose a picture from a magazine, and the model was wearing clothing they would like to wear, too. The picture reminded them of their goal.

Many different types of behavior are modified or triggered with a reminder mechanism. Posting slogans around an office serves as a reminder to workers to put the customer first and are often added when a new customer service program is launched. Or people put a rubber band around their wrist to remind them to make an important call. Some people carry a symbolic reminder, such as a stone or a small note to themselves, in their pockets or handbags. They could be reminding themselves about a wide variety of things, from keeping their tempers with their children to taking deep breaths and relaxing instead of doing every task in a rushed way. I once heard of a woman who carried a picture of Mahatma Gandhi in her wallet to remind her to keep a peaceful attitude!

The inhalers work in a similar way. The presence of an inhaler is a reminder to use it instead of eating. Seeing it, touching it, and sniffing it are all part of the reminder mechanism. We don't specifically recommend food diaries and prefer that our patients keep a journal instead, but some people find that keeping a food diary prompts them to eat less. If you must actually write down the food you ate that day, eating becomes a conscious act rather than an un-conscious one. In a similar way, the inhaler works to make reaching for food a conscious act. Reaching for an inhaler gives you enough time to determine if you're really hungry or if you're just accustomed to eating something sweet at 3:00 P.M.

Or, some people might feel hungry, but they decide that being overweight is worse than an occasional hunger pang. They reach for the inhaler, the odor stimulates the satiety center, and more than one mechanism comes into play.

Reminders tend to act on the left side of the brain, the cognitive or intellectual center. The little id starts saying, "I want, I want, I want," but if you use the inhaler as a reminder mechanism, the rational brain takes over and says, "Not now, you aren't even hungry," or, "You just ate lunch, you don't need more food." In other words, the odor device is able to inhibit the limbic drives and allows the rational self to take over. We're not making judgments about the limbic brain, with all its built-in drives. We're just taming it, as we do in many other areas of life, from sex to sleeping patterns.

I'm Feeling So Good

Earlier in the book, I discussed studies showing that certain odors can reduce different types of anxiety. It's certainly possible that the odors work in controlling food intake because they also may reduce anxiety and produce an enhanced sense of well-being.

Many people eat when they're anxious—although it's also true that some people lose their appetite when their anxiety level is high. For now, I'm generalizing and saying that overweight people are probably among the group that eats more and probably eats faster in anxiety-provoking situations. And this anxiety doesn't have to be over huge events or dire circumstances. Being anxious about a big test or meeting a new client or having a first date are all situations that provoke anxiety. Many a bride or groom has vowed to lose weight before the big wedding, and for several months they succeed in losing some pounds. But as the day draws closer, they become anxious about the details and perhaps even the big step they're taking, and they begin eating more. It's not really such a mystery when we understand that emotions affect all types of behavior.

Odors may both reduce anxiety and increase well-being. When we feel relaxed and cheerful, we feel better about ourselves, which in turn reduces the need to eat whatever food is handy to feel secure. The inhalers may act like a security blanket, and the urge to eat dissipates.

Nostalgia, Or the Sweet Odors of Youth

We know that an odor is the fastest way to trigger nostalgic reverie. A whiff of a particular scent can bring back entire scenes from the past, and you've no doubt had this experience. The scent of a certain cologne reminds you of your grandmother, and in a matter of seconds, you're recalling events and scenes that took place, depending on your age, ten, twenty, fifty, or even sixty or seventy years ago. If other people are around, you might start telling a story from that time gone by, and if you're alone, you might spend several minutes in a daydream-like state.

Most people recall pleasant events from the past in the presence of a particular scent, but in some cases—veterans, for example—the smell of burning gasoline or rubber is enough to evoke extreme anxiety or even panic. It's as if they are for that moment back on the scene of the battle. This is not uncommon among men and women who have been diagnosed with Post Traumatic Stress Disorder (PTSD).

We once conducted a study in which we asked close to one thousand people of all ages, coming from forty-five states and thirty-nine countries, to name the number one odor that made them nostalgic for their childhoods. The smell of baked goods was the primary odor mentioned, which shows how closely food and childhood memories are linked. The other choices depended largely on where people were raised. Those from the East Coast named the smell of flowers as the most powerful nostalgic odor, while those from the South told us that the smell of fresh air took them back to childhood every time. Mid-westerners mentioned the odor of farm animals, and those from the West Coast named the odor of barbecued meat—a pair of smells that we could call "before and after" odors.

Country of origin made a difference, too. People raised in some of the African countries mentioned the smell of maize, while their Scandinavian counterparts spoke of herring, the latter being proof that no universally agreed-upon list of good and bad smells exists. Likewise, age was an important factor. Older people, those born before 1930, were more likely to mention natural smells—meadows, pine trees, hay, and so forth. But those born later, especially people born after 1950, were more likely to describe artificial smells, from Play-Doh™ to plastic. (What these changes tell us about our society and particularly about the future of environmental concerns is an important issue, but a subject for another book.)

We can speculate that the odors available in inhalers today may increase a sense of well-being because they trigger what we call an olfactory-evoked nostalgic response. Just as the scents might reduce anxiety, the odors might trigger recall of pleasant times. An odor doesn't need to be the number one favorite to induce warm feelings and memories of happier times. We may not be conscious of our responses either. A strawberry odor or a whiff of a banana inhaler may bring about pleasant feelings and even trigger a memory, and we don't have the slightest idea why. This is not unusual. We do know, however, that many study subjects said that using the odors made them feel good.

This Isn't Where It's Supposed to Be, So I Don't Like It

It's possible that the odors reduce appetite because they are what we call "contextually discordant" odors. What do I mean by that? An odor must be perceived as matching a context or it causes us to view it negatively. If we smell fish in a movie theater instead of popcorn, we might say there's a bad smell, and we might leave. The same fish served on a terrace in the Caribbean is an inviting smell—if you enjoy fish in the first place.

Mark Twain wrote a short story called "The Invalid's Story," in which a hobo hops on a train car in which there is what he perceives to be a coffin containing a rotting body. The stench is overwhelming, and eventually, he can no longer stand it. He jumps off the train and lands in a snow bank, and ultimately he develops pneumonia. When he's found, he is taken to a hospital, where because of his grave condition, he's expected to die shortly. For his last meal, he is given a piece of cheese that came from the crate that he had thought was a coffin containing a rotting body. In other words, an odor that is appreciated in one setting is disliked if the context isn't correct. Had the hobo recognized the "bad" smell as cheese, he might have had a feast.

For some people, the smell of sausage pizza is tempting at lunchtime but can be sickening first thing in the morning. The odor devices may keep people from eating because the inhaler is sometimes used in a context where no food is expected to be around. The odor is out of place and, therefore, reduces hunger.

Context aside, we and others have thought that a bad smell would logically reduce the urge to eat, but this turns out not to be the case. Aversion therapy tends not to work because people have a natural tendency to avoid it. If you're asked to sniff an odor that nauseates you, you might try it for a day or two, but you would rather eat than sniff bad odors all day long.

Choose the odors, both food and nonfood specific, that you like, and you will use them more often. If you start with the idea that you'll choose to sniff unpleasant smells, the odor program likely will not work for you.

The Tip of the Iceberg Is at the Tip of Your Nose

If you decide to use odors to reduce or control your weight, you are participating in the tip of the iceberg of research on our precious and vital sense of smell. In the next decade or two, odors will be increasingly used in health-care environments, commercial settings, schools, and workplaces. The Japanese and others are conducting research, too, and one day we'll probably use odors to help us wake up in the morning, work more efficiently during the day, exercise vigorously after work, feel romantic in the evening, and sleep well at night. And right in there in the mix are the odors we'll use to control appetite and reduce or maintain weight. If anyone tells you this is just another diet scheme, show this book to that person. Once the validity of odors becomes widely recognized, there may never be another weight loss diet created again—and that's good news.

Ask Away! The Most Common Questions about Odors and Weight Loss

1. You seem to be quite concerned about women and body image issues. But isn't it true that thinner is better?

You're right, I am concerned about the emphasis on a particular ideal body image in our society, one that is especially cruel to women. The range of healthful weight is much larger than once believed, and the extreme thinness that is promoted today is harmful in many ways, but primarily emotionally. It has led to an increase in anorexia nervosa among young women and even some men. When we have more than 50 percent of grade school girls tell researchers that they're on diets, something is seriously wrong. Men, but especially women, sometimes reach normal weight but still feel fat. They feel that way because they still don't look like the models in clothing ads or like famous Hollywood stars. The fact is that many of those stars have body doubles—so even they don't fit the impossible ideal. This situation is bad enough for adult women, but it's devastating for young girls and teenagers.

2. You seem to talk about eating in restaurants a lot, but isn't it better to eat at home as much as possible?

One could make an argument that if we all ate more home-cooked meals, we would have a more healthful diet. (One could make the argument the other way, too, depending on the amount and kind of food we're eating at home.) However, diets that advise cooking at home go against a major trend and make it more difficult to stick to a prescribed food plan. The vast majority of people eat *at least* one meal in a restaurant or office or school cafeteria every day. Many people eat two meals away from home every day. I prefer to work with reality as it exists, rather than give recommendations based on ideal situations that *could* exist if we all changed our lifestyles. Those recommendations are usually too difficult to follow, and feelings of failure and deprivation result.

Most of our study subjects continued eating many meals a week in restaurants, but they used the odor devices and were able to leave food on the plate or take it home in a doggy bag. Restaurants are not automatically places to overeat. Remember, people often cook big meals and consume every scrap. The odor devices help people eat less in every setting.

3. I have allergies, but not asthma. Could the odors harm me?

Common allergies to pollen and so forth are not likely to interfere with the use of the odors, except if the nasal passages are completely stuffed up and the ability to smell is temporarily gone. No one has ever reported nasal irritation, so we have to assume that if allergies aren't interfering with detecting the odors, the devices are safe. If you are concerned, however, check with your doctor. To date, the only people who should not use these devices are those with asthma and those who have migraine headaches that are triggered by odors.

4. I'm a vegetarian. Will the odors work just as well for me?

Absolutely. Contrary to popular opinion, there are overweight vegetarians, although admittedly, they are fewer in number than their carnivorous brothers and sisters. I've spoken with many vegetarians with a strong "sweet tooth," and they found the scales inching up, despite their grain, bean, and vegetable-based diets. My recommendation is to use odors regardless of how you define your diet.

5. Are you sure I won't become addicted to the inhaler?

You may miss the inhaler if you forget it; you may feel as if you are dependent on it, which at first is a good thing; you may find that others are concerned about how much you're sniffing. However, this is not the same as a harmful addiction, as addiction is scientifically defined. Using the odor device becomes habitual, and when and if you want to, you can stop using it. You'll break a habit, not a chemical dependency. I predict, however, that odor devices are tools we can use for long-term weight control in our society. With the abundance of food we have and the constant food messages, obesity will probably be a continuing problem, and the odor program is a way to combat it safely and effectively.

6. My sense of smell isn't very good. Will the odors work for me or should I abandon the idea of losing weight with this method?

Those whose sense of smell falls into the normal range to above-normal range lose weight faster than those whose sense of smell is below normal. But unless your sense of smell is essentially gone, which means you suffer from a condition kown as anosmia, you will still receive some benefit from the odors. You will lose weight more slowly than those with better ability to smell, but I encourage you to go ahead and give the odors a try.

7. Are the odor devices safe for my children and teenagers?

So far, the odor devices have been shown to be safe, except for people with asthma and for those whose migraine headaches can be triggered by an odor. However, using the odors for weight loss has been tested only on people age eighteen and older. I can't tell you if the odors are effective for children. My concern about children using the device is that they will use it when they don't need it, in their ongoing attempts to become too thin. I would proceed with caution, particularly if weight is only a vanity issue.

8. I would like to lose 5, maybe 10 pounds. Are the devices good for minor weight problems?

The devices can be used for weight control and weight loss. The number of pounds doesn't matter. I suggest using them moderately and losing those few pounds slowly. I don't condone using the devices for a week or two just to fit into a certain piece of clothing or for a special occasion—they are not meant to be used for crash dieting. Besides, weight that is lost very quickly tends to be regained. Another question, of course, is how many people really need to lose 5 or 10 pounds? In my experience, exercise that tones the body is probably better in the long run than trying to take off 5 pounds by restricting one's diet.

9. Are you sure that the odors won't hurt my nasal passages?

We have no reports of any difficulty with the nasal passages. These are odors, not medications or drugs. We occasionally received a call from a person who put the inhaler into the nose, rather than simply holding it under the nose. So, if there is a caution, that's it. Be sure to keep the inhaler outside the nose, not in it.

10. Will the odors ruin my appetite? I was on one diet where my appetite all but disappeared. I began to feel sick at the sight of food, and it was frightening. Naturally, I went off the diet. Is there any chance this could happen with this program?

We have never heard anyone tell us that their appetite disappeared, even among those people who sniffed more than three hundred times a day. We respect your appetite and want you only to eat less of what you usually eat. Aversion therapy doesn't work anyway. As you said, you stopped the diet when your appetite became poor. You were right to be afraid of such a diet.

11. Will I just gradually reduce the amount of sniffing I do when I reach my goal weight?

Yes, that's what happens. You can use the device to help maintain a good weight for you. You will probably use it less, but you know it is there. Some patients find the devices help them keep the good eating habits they've developed. In fact, we recommend that people who have struggled with weight all their lives consider the odor program one they can use safely for a lifetime.

12. The odors that are available for weight loss purposes are artificial-manufactured-smells. Are they really as good as the natural odors I find in the specialty shops?

The world is filled with artificial odors. The lemon scent in your dish soap is artificial, as is the strawberry flavor in soft drinks and powdered drinks. The odors in popular candies, such as jelly beans, peppermint, or licorice, are also manufactured smells. The list goes on and on.

The odors found in specialty shops, recommended by aromatherapy books, are derived from plant sources, although they are generally not food odors. They are pleasant, and if you like them, go ahead and use them in your home. Jasmine, peppermint, lavender, sandalwood, oil of rose, lemon, and so forth are available in both natural and manufactured form.

When we research the effects of odors, we always use manufactured scents, not only because they are less expensive to produce, but because the concentration of the odorant can be controlled and made uniform. The natural scents tend be unstable, in that concentrations vary from plant to plant and even hour to hour in the same plant.

So far, we have no evidence that the brain distinguishes between a manufactured odor and a natural one.

• • •

For the vast majority of people, the odor program is safe and effective. The most important advice I offer you now is to *get started*. Don't worry about calories or fat grams. Enjoy your food—and observe yourself eating less of it. Begin to move around and add some exercise, and the pounds will melt away.

I want you to enjoy the odor experience—and I wish you the best in your quest to achieve a healthful weight.

Appendix

Weight Reduction through Inhalation of Odorants
A.R. HIRSCH, M.D.,[1] and R. Gomez[2]

ABSTRACT Despite the pervasive problem of obesity and the expenditure of billions of dollars devising methods of losing weight, no studies have been published on the role of the olfactory sense in determining weight. To assess the effect of inhalation of certain aromas upon weight control, we studied 3193 overweight volunteers. Their average age was 43 years, average height 65 inches, and average weight 217 pounds. Each was given an inhaler containing a blend of odorants and instructed to inhale three times in each nostril whenever feeling hungry. New inhalers containing a new blend of odorants were supplied each month over a period of 6 months. Those subjects whose test scores showed they had good olfactory abilities and who use their inhalers frequently, ate 2 to 4 meals a day, felt bad about overeating, but did not feel bad about themselves lost nearly 5 pounds, or 2% of body weight per month. It appears possible that inhalation of certain aromas can induce sustained weight loss over a 6-month period.

KEY WORDS Obesity, Smell, Weight reduction

[1] *Smell and Taste Treatment and Research Foundation, Ltd., Water Tower Place, Suite 990W, 845 North Michigan Avenue, Chicago, IL 60611, USA*

[2] *University of Illinois Medical School, Chicago, IL 60612, USA*

Introduction

With a third to a quarter of the American population over-weight, obesity is rampant in contemporary society. At any given time, 40% of women and 24% of men are trying to lose weight and of these, 84% of women and 76–78% of men are dieting for this purpose. In the USA, losing weight has become a national obsession. Furthermore, over 30 billion dollars are spent each year devising a plethora of new diets and methods for losing weight, many of which are ineffective.[1]

States of hunger and satiety are known to be of crucial importance in the regulation of weight, and the perception of hunger is multivariant; environmental stimuli, psychological substrate, and internal physiology all contribute a share. Everyday experiences attest to the influence of ambient aromas on our appetites; we salivate at the smell of freshly baked cookies and feel nauseated at a whiff of sewer gas. When we are hungry, foods smell better and therefore taste better. Conversely, olfactory ability wanes when we are satisfied, lessening the hedonics of further gustation.[2]

Anatomic connections of the olfactory bulb to the ven-tromedial nucleus of the hypothalamus, the satiety center, authenticate these observations,[3] as does the presence of cholecystokinin, a gastric satiety factor, as a neurotransmitter in the olfactory bulb.[4] The fact that patients with acute anosmia often gain weight suggests that a failure of the olfactory-satiety feedback mechanism may be involved.[5]

Thus it is perhaps surprising, that amid the proliferating studies of weight regulation, no reports have been published assessing the role of olfaction. The purpose of our investi-gation was to explore the effect of odors in regulating body weight—specifically, to determine whether inhaling certain sweet aromas would facilitate weight loss in overweight subjects.

Materials and Methods

SUBJECTS We selected 3193 volunteers for this study who were at least 10 pounds overweight, between the ages of 18 and 64 years, had no history of asthma, were not pregnant, breast-feeding or planning to become pregnant during the 6-month period of the study.

PROCEDURE Subjects were given inhalers containing blends of aromatic ingredients and instructed to inhale three times in each nostril whenever hungry. They were told not to deviate from their usual diet and exercise habits. Then each month for a period of 6 months, the subjects were given new inhalers containing a new aromatic blend in a sequence of peppermint, banana, and green apple. Subjects were weighted monthly.

INSTRUMENTS Subjects' olfactory abilities were measured using the Chicago Smell Test[6] and the thiophane-odor-threshold test of Amoore.[7] Odor hedonics were rated using a visual analog scale. All subjects completed demographic questionnaires and psychological tests, Beck Depression Inventory,[8] and Zung Depression Scales.[9]

STATISTICAL ANALYSIS Data were analyzed using Pearson Correlation coefficients and I tests for the difference of two proportions.

Results

SUBJECT POPULATION A typical volunteer subject was a 43-year-old white woman, about 5'5" tall with a medium-sized frame, weighing 217 pounds and whose ideal weight was 129 pounds. She was a Catholic separated from her husband and either an unskilled worker or unemployed. She exercised 9 minutes a day, used alcohol moderately, and did not smoke or use drugs.

Table 1. Physical characteristics

	% of Subjects (n = 3193)
SEX	
Female	86.4%
Male	13.6%
FRAME SIZE	
Small	11.9%
Medium	57.9%
Large	30.2%
RACE	
White	67.9%
Black	25.4%
Hispanic	4.6%
	Average
Age	42.9 yrs
Height	64.7 in
Initial Weight	216.9 lbs
Ideal weight*	129.0 lbs

Based on basal metabolism index.

Table 2. Social characteristics

	% of Subjects (n = 3193)
MARITAL STATUS	
Separated	44.5%
Single	23.2%
Divorced	15.4%
Married	13.3%
EMPLOYMENT STATUS	
Unskilled or unemployed	75.0%
Skilled workers	25.0%
RELIGION	
Catholic	48.8%
Jewish	7.0%
Protestant	6.8%

The group was predominantly female—86.4% female and 13.6% male. Physical characteristics are shown in Table 1. Three quarters of the subjects were unskilled workers or unemployed. Only 13% were married. Social characteristics are shown in Table 2.

Slightly more than half the subjects exercised and their average time spent exercising was 9 minutes per day. Most of the group used alcohol moderately, about one quarter smoked, and one fifth used diet pills. Nine percent used sleeping pills and almost 10% used other nonprescription drugs. Behavioral traits are shown in Table 3.

Slightly over half the subject population consumed three meals a day; almost a third ate fewer than three meals a day.

Table 3. Behavioral Traits

	% of Subjects (n = 3193)
Exercised	50.9%
Smoked	25.1%
Daily	17.7%
Used alcohol	72.1%
Daily	4.3%
Weekly	17.6%
Monthly	15.9%
Less	4.3%
Used drugs	
Diet pills	20.6%
Daily	1.8%
Sleeping pills	9.2%
Daily or weekly	2.5%
Tranquilizers	6.6%
Daily	1.5%
Marijuana	4.3%
Amphetamines	0.4%
Daily	0.5%
Cocaine	1.6%
Daily	0.4%
Other nonprescription drugs	9.8%

Over a third had four to nine snacks a day. Almost all liked chocolate. Almost half were subject to binge eating and over half craved certain foods. Almost 80% said they ate more when they were nervous. The eating behavior of those in the study is shown in Table 4.

Table 4. Eating behavior and food preferences

	% of Subjects (n = 3193)
No. of meals/day	
< 3	31.7%
3	54.3%
4-9	14.0%
Snacks/day	
4-9	35.5%
3	30.8%
0	0.5%
Like chocolate	98.9%
Eat 5 or more chocolate bars/wk	54.7%
Eat 5 or more bananas/wk	9.3%
Eat 1-5 ice cream bars/wk	29.3%
Eat 1-5 apples/wk	76.4%
Eat 1-5 mint candies/wk	48.4%
Binge eating	48.7%
Favorite binge foods:	
Chocolate	12.8%
Potato chips	9.6%
Candy	7.7%
Ice cream	6.0%
Pretzels	3.3%
Crave certain foods	55.9%
Chocolate	15.6%
Candy	6.7%
Potato chips	4.6%
Ice cream	3.8%
Pretzels	3.1%
Fast frequently to control weight	14.1%
Diet currently	16.7%
Eat more when nervous	79.4%

Table 5. Psychological factors upon admission into this study

	% of Subjects (n = 3193)
Complained of impaired sex life due to overweight	89.9%
Felt bad about overeating	78.3%
Were too tired to do almost anything	76.0%
Perceived themselves as unattractive or ugly	76.0%
Hated themselves	56.1%
Became irritated more easily than usual	54.8%
Worried about physical health	53.4%
Felt dissatisfied with their lives	52.9%
Criticized or blamed themselves for everything bad that happened to them	47.7%
Lost some or all interest in sex	46.7%
Felt sad most or all of the time	34.6%
Had trouble making decisions	34.3%
Felt guilty much or most of the time	33.7%
Had lost interest in other people	31.7%
Avoided others because of eating problems	29.7%
Cried more than usual or wanted to cry but could not	24.0%
Had times of feeling a failure	22.7%
Had given up hope of losing weight	20.4%
Felt discouraged about the future	20.1%
Felt punished	15.2%
Had no pleasure other than those revolving around food	10.8%
Wished for suicide	8.0%

Psychological difficulties were prominent among our subjects. Impaired sex life, bad feelings about overeating, fatigue, and poor self-image were very common with more than three quarters of the subjects so affected. Over half the subjects said they hated themselves. Indecisiveness, guilt feelings, and loss of interest in others affected about a third of the group. Eight percent said they wished for suicide. Psychological factors upon admission into the study are shown in Table 5.

Table 6. History of overweight and its effects

	% of Subjects (n = 3193)
Had been in diet or obesity programs	51.0%
with M.D.s	23.5%
with Weight Watchers	27.6%
with Office-based centers	22.2%
Suffered effects of overweight	
Medical problems	15.7%
Previously diagnosed bulimia	0.7%
Previously diagnosed anorexia nervosa	0.3%
Family disharmony	89.0%
Insomnia	50.4%
Trouble working	54.2%
Had obese mothers	45.4%
Had obese fathers	26.7%
	No. of married subjects (n = 425)
Had obese spouses	79.2%

The age of onset of weight problems averaged 20.8 years for our subjects, and ranged from birth to 63 years. Slightly over half of those in the group had been in one or more of 66 different diet or obesity programs. Many subjects reported suffering various effects of overweight. Most frequently mentioned was family disharmony, with 89% of the study population naming this problem. Over half the subjects suffered from insomnia and had trouble working as a result of being overweight. Table 6 shows the history of obesity and its effects among those in our study.

Many subjects had obese parents: 45% had obese mothers, who averaged 45.4 pounds overweight; about 27% had obese fathers, who averaged 40.6 pounds overweight. Of those who were married (425 subjects), 79.2% had obese spouses, who averaged 38.6 pounds overweight (Table 6).

Olfactory Status

Most subjects were able to detect the three odorants in the Chicago Smell Test, namely banana, apple, and mint, and to correctly identify at least one of the three. On Amoore's odor threshold test for thiophane, 85% of our subjects had a threshold within the normal range of -25 to +25 decismels; 15% of subjects had a threshold of 55 decismels indicating hyposmia (Table 7).

Table 7. Olfactory status

	% of Subjects able to	
	Detect	Identify
Chicago Smell Test*		
Banana	99.0%	15.8%
Apple	98.3%	16.9%
Mint	99.5%	76.0%
Amoore's Threshold Test**		
Thiophane		
-25 decismels	0.0%	
0 decismels	12.8%	
25 decismels	72.2%	
55 decismels	15.0%	

Normal subjects are able to detect all three odors and to identify at least one.

**Normal range is -25 to +25 decismels.*

USE OF INHALERS Frequency of use of inhalers varied from three times a day (three sniffs in each nostril each time = 18 sniffs) to 48 times a day (288 sniffs).

WEIGHT LOSS The amount of weight the subjects lost directly correlated with the frequency of their use of the inhalers ($p < 0.002$). Those who showed good olfactory ability, that is, a threshold of 0–25 decismels in Amoore's thiophane test, who correctly identified the apple odorant in the

Chicago Smell Test, who ate an average of two to four meals a day and felt bad about overeating but did not feel bad about themselves, experienced an average weight reduction of 4.7 pounds, or 2.1% of body weight per month. Individuals lost up to 18 pounds per month. Other characteristics that correlated with weight loss were medium or large frame size, not avoiding others, eating fewer chocolate bars, eating more apples, and eating more mint candies. The characteristics that correlate with weight loss and their p values are shown in Table 8.

Table 8. Characteristics that correlate with weight loss

Frequency of inhaler use	$p < 0.002$
Amoore's thiophane threshold 0-25 decismels	$p < 0.050$
Chicago Smell Test —ability to identify apple odor	$p < 0.050$
Medium or large frame size	$p < 0.020$
Not avoiding others	$p < 0.005$
Not feeling bad about oneself	$p < 0.005$
Liking chocolate	$p < 0.008$
Eating fewer chocolate bars	$p < 0.040$
Eating more apples	$p < 0.060$
Eating more mint candies	$p < 0.060$

Subjects who showed poor olfactory abilities, those who tended to snack more than five times a day, and those who disliked chocolate did not lose weight.

Conclusion

These data suggest that it may be possible for individuals with good olfaction, by inhaling certain aromas, to induce and sustain loss of weight over a 6-month period. Theoretically, this approach may be helpful for use in connection with a program of nutrition and exercise to facilitate weight reduction.

References

1. NIH Technology Assessment Conference Panel. Methods for voluntary weight loss and control. Ann Intern Med 1992; 116:942-949

2. Hirsch AR. Demography in olfaction. *Proc Inst Med Chgo* 1992; 45:6

3. Brodal A. *Neurological anatomy in relation to clinical medicine*, 3rd ed. New York: Oxford University Press, 1981; 653, 751

4. Greer CA. Structural organization of the olfactory system. In: Getchell TV, Doty TL, Bartoshuk LM, Snow JB, (eds). *Smell and taste in health and disease*. New York: Raven Press, 1991; 78

5. Hirsch AR, Dougherty DD. Inhalation of 2-acetylpyridine for weight reduction. *Chem Senses* 1993; 18-570

6. Hirsch AR, Cain DR. Evaluation of the Chicago smell test in a normal population. *Chem Senses* 1992; 17:642-643

7. Amoore J, Ollman B. Practical test kits for quantitatively evaluating the sense of smell. *Rhinology* 1983; 21:49-54

8. Beck AT, Ward C, Mendelson M, et al. Inventory for measuring depression. *Arch Gen Psych* 1961; 4:561-571

9. Zung WWK. Self-rating depression scale. *Arch Gen Psych* 1965; 12:63-70

Reprinted by permission of the *Journal of Neurological and Orthopedic Medicine and Surgery* (1995) 16: 26–31.